T0252860

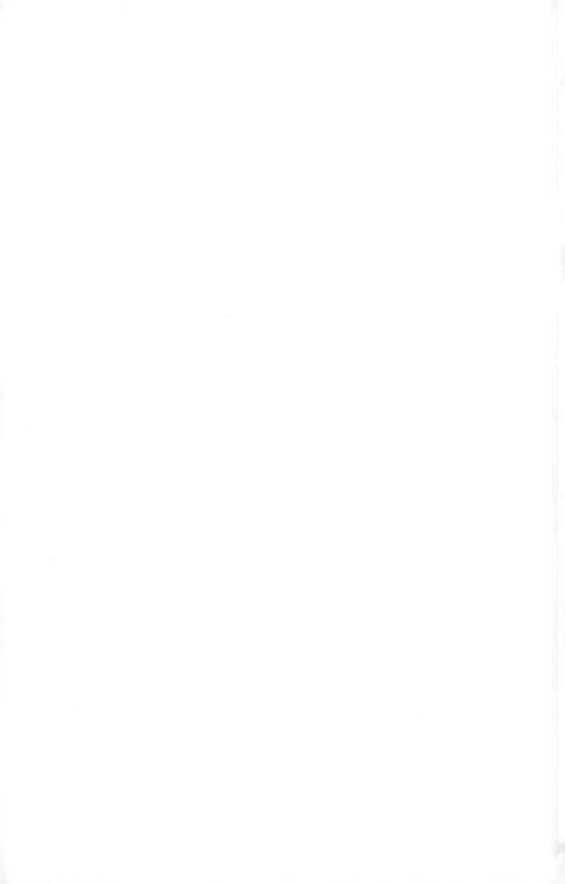

MENTAL HEALTH SERVICES AND COMMUNITY CARE
A Critical History

Ian Cummins

First published in Great Britain in 2020 by

Policy Press
University of Bristol
1-9 Old Park Hill
Bristol
BS2 8BB
UK
t: +44 (0)117 954 5940
pp-info@bristol.ac.uk
www.policypress.co.uk

North America office:
Policy Press
c/o The University of Chicago Press
1427 East 60th Street
Chicago, IL 60637, USA
t: +1 773 702 7700
f: +1 773-702-9756
sales@press.uchicago.edu
www.press.uchicago.edu

© Policy Press 2020

British Library Cataloguing in Publication Data
A catalogue record for this book is available from the British Library

Library of Congress Cataloging-in-Publication Data
A catalog record for this book has been requested

ISBN 978-1-4473-5059-0 (hardback)
ISBN 978-1-4473-5063-7 (ePDF)
ISBN 978-1-4473-5064-4 (ePub)

The right of Ian Cummins to be identified as the author of this work has been
asserted by him in accordance with the Copyright, Designs and Patents Act 1988.

All rights reserved: no part of this publication may be reproduced, stored in a retrieval system,
or transmitted in any form or by any means, electronic, mechanical, photocopying, recording,
or otherwise without the prior permission of Policy Press.

The statements and opinions contained within this publication are solely those of the author
and not of the University of Bristol or Policy Press. The University of Bristol and Policy
Press disclaim responsibility for any injury to persons or property resulting from any material
published in this publication.

Policy Press works to counter discrimination on grounds of gender, race,
disability, age and sexuality.

Cover design by Robin Hawes
Front cover image: Alamy stock images, J9E16Y
Printed and bound in Great Britain by CPI Group (UK) Ltd,
Croydon, CR0 4YY
Policy Press uses environmentally responsible print partners

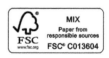

In memory of Dr Jo Milner (1960–2018)

My PhD supervisor Dr Jo Milner died in December
2018. I owe her a huge personal and professional debt.
Jo was wonderfully supportive friend and colleague.
Without her I would never have overcome the barriers
to completing my thesis. She was committed to
challenging injustice, inequality and discrimination
in all forms wherever she encountered it. She was a
supporter of the work of Freedom from Torture
(www.freedomfromtorture.org/)
This book is dedicated, with love, to her memory.

Into the nothingness of scorn and noise,
Into the living sea of waking dreams,
Where there is neither sense of life or joys,
But the vast shipwreck of my life's esteems;
Even the dearest that I loved the best
Are strange—nay, rather, stranger than the rest.

John Clare, 'I Am'

Contents

About the author

Ian Cummins qualified as a probation officer and subsequently worked as a mental health social worker. His research interests in the criminal justice system and the history of mental health services reflect his practice experience. He has previously published *Poverty, Inequality and Social Work: The Impact of Neo-liberalism and Austerity Politics on Welfare Provision* with Policy Press in 2018 and *Mental Health Social Work Reimagined* with Policy Press in 2019.

Acknowledgements

My late mother worked incredibly hard to enable me to continue my education and take advantage of the opportunities that it offered. She passed on her love of books to me. I hope that she would have enjoyed this one. I owe a huge debt to my brother and my sisters for their love and support.

I would like to thank Isobel Bainton, Shannon Kneis and all the staff at Policy Press who have been unfailing supportive of this and other projects that I have undertaken. I am very grateful to the anonymous reviewers of the initial proposal and drafts of the book for their time and constructive suggestions. I am, of course, responsible for any failings, admissions or errors in the final version.

I regard myself as extremely lucky to have had the wonderful support and encouragement of colleagues and friends: Janet Chapman, Elizabeth Collier, David Edmondson, Akwugo Emejulu, Paul Michael Garrett, Maria Grant, Marian Foley, Jameel Hadi, Stephen Jones, Emma Kelly, Gavin Kendall, Martin King, Karen Kinghorn, Jane Lucas, David McKendrick, Bernard Melling, Lisa Morriss, Muzammil Quraishi, Kate Parkinson, Donna Peach, David Platten, Nick Platten, Sarah Pollock, Barry Schilling, Jonathan Simon, Imogen Tyler, Joanne Warner, Stephen Webb, Joanne Westwood, Toni Woods.

I am extremely grateful to Gavin Davidson, Hester Parr and Cheryl McGeachan all of whom took the time to read a draft of the book.

I completed this project during a period of study leave. I am grateful for the School of Health and Society at Salford for facilitating this. I would particularly like to thank Professor Joanne Westwood, who was very supportive of my initial application.

I have also enjoyed virtual support from @asifamhp, @SchrebersSister and @Mental_Elf

Most importantly of all, I would not have been able to complete this work without my wife, Marilyn, my sons, Elliot and Nelson, and his partner, Eilidh.

Introduction

When Theresa May became Prime Minister in July 2016, she made a speech on the steps of Downing Street in which she outlined a series of 'burning injustices' her administration would seek to tackle. Many were struck by the irony of this commitment to tackling inequality and disadvantages coming, as it did, from a senior member of the coalition and Conservative governments that since 2010 had introduced a series of policies which had targeted those living in poverty and the most vulnerable. The scandals of the revelation of the real impact of the 'hostile environment' created by May's Home Office and the appalling treatment of the Windrush generation lay ahead. In May 2017, May announced that a review would be undertaken of the 'flawed' Mental Health Act (MHA). In making the announcement she stated:

> 'On my first day in Downing Street last July, I described shortfalls in mental health services as one of the burning injustices in our country. It is abundantly clear to me that the discriminatory use of a law passed more than three decades ago is a key part of the reason for this. So today I am pledging to rip up the 1983 Act and introduce in its place a new law which finally confronts the discrimination and unnecessary detention that takes place too often.' (Savage, 2017)

It was later announced that the MHA review would be chaired by an eminent psychiatrist, Sir Simon Wessely. The review was completed in December 2018 (Department of Health and Social Care, 2018). Its recommendations are discussed in the final chapter of this book. In his foreword to the final report, Sir Simon outlines the case for change. The increase in the number of detentions – formal admissions using the powers of the MHA – was one of the factors highlighted. This is not a new issue. The process and rates of detention under the MHA, coupled with the conditions on wards and patients' negative experiences have been long standing issues. The review also examined an issue that has long been a scar on modern mental health services: over-representation of people from black and minority ethnic (BAME) groups among patients detained under the MHA. Finally, there were concerns that the current mental health legislation in England and Wales did not comply with international standards on human rights.

The issues that the Wessely review was asked to consider are not new. They have appeared at various points, perhaps in slightly different configurations over the past 50 to 60 years. This is the period of deinstitutionalisation – the closure programme of long stay mental hospitals that was announced in Enoch Powell's Water Tower speech in 1961. Despite their closure, these Gothic decaying institutions have cast a long shadow over mental health services. This volume examines the policy of community care that followed deinstitutionalisation. Community care is used as a shorthand for a range of community based mental health and other welfare services that support those experiencing mental distress. I should note here that terminology in the field of mental health is a problematic area. I use a range of terms in this volume: mad, the mentally ill, service user, people with mental health problems. This is not laziness or sloppiness on my part. The terms have all been and continue to be used in popular and academic discourse. I am not aware that there is a term that is widely accepted or not seen as problematic in some way. The terms reflect underlying values. I accept that some of these terms might be offensive. I apologise in advance for any offence caused to readers. This was not my intention.

The volume presents a critical history of deinstitutionalisation and the subsequent policy of community care. This, of course, points to one of the major criticisms of the policies. One should not have replaced the other, they should have gone hand in hand. In developing this analysis, I have been influenced by Rose's model of a 'history of the present' (Rose, 1994: 53). This requires an investigation 'from the point of view of a problem that concerns one today, the diverse connections and liaisons that have brought it into existence and given its saliency and its characteristics'. As part of this process, the current and historical 'practices of truth situate persons in particular relations of force' are analysed.

Chapter 1 provides a short introduction to deinstitutionalisation and community care, outlining the fiscal and ideological drivers of the reforms. The following chapter uses critical notions of space and place to explore the meaning and values attached to the terms 'asylum' and 'community'. It argues that reductionist binary notions that present the community as an inherently progressive alternative to the asylum proved at best optimistic, at worst naive. Community care was introduced at a time when the impact of neoliberal economic and social policies was doing huge damage to the structure of local communities. The book then focuses on the development of mental health policy in the late 1980s and the early 1990s, outlining the way the pressures on mental health services developed. It examines the way that a series of high profile crimes committed by people with serious mental health issues and the subsequent inquiries led to call for reforms of the MHA. The period of deinstitutionalisation has been accompanied by a huge expansion of the use of imprisonment. Chapter 4 discusses the way that the penal state has become, in many circumstances, a de facto provider of mental health care. The reforms of the MHA and the introduction of Community Treatment Orders (CTOs) are then discussed. I argue that the introduction of the CTO marks the end of an official commitment to 'community care'. Deinstitutionalisation is a policy that has been adopted in the majority countries in the world. Examples of its impact are discussed. The final chapters examine the landscape of contemporary mental health services.

2

Community care: a brief overview

Introduction

This short chapter provides a brief overview of the development of community care. It examines the way that the asylum became an obsolete institution – certainly one that had few defenders in the early 1980s. In giving a brief overview of the intellectual underpinnings of community care, the chapter introduces a series of issues – deinstitutionalisation and the penal state, community care inquiries and the asylum/community binary – which are examined in depth in subsequent chapters. Community care is a complex and highly influential shift in mental health services. As with all policies, there were a series of drivers behind the policy. I would summarise these as a combination of progressive idealism that attacked the whole notion that institutions could ever provide humane, dignified care and fiscal conservatism. Progressive idealism and fiscal conservatism are unlikely and uneasy bedfellows. The result was a policy that was imbued with service user rights but was introduced at a time of welfare retrenchment. In the UK and the US, this major shift to a community oriented vision of mental health service provision was introduced by governments committed to a small state and convinced of the supremacy of the market.

Community care is a phrase that does not appear in many, if any, contemporary mental health policy documents. It has either been discarded or is so deeply embedded that it is not worth commenting on. One of the aims of this volume is to examine the reasons behind the disappearance of community care from official discourse. The closure of the large psychiatric hospitals that had been built in the 19th century is one of the most significant social policies of the last 50 years. The process of asylum closure is usually referred to as *deinstitutionalisation*. Estroff (1981) identified four groups of patients who were affected by the process of deinstitutionalisation:

- long-term hospital patients who were discharged;
- patients who experienced potentially multiple psychotic episodes and hospital admissions – this group was treated as outpatients or with short, crisis-oriented admissions;

- patients who were treated on an outpatient basis;
- those patients who experienced a first serious episode of mental distress and were not admitted to hospital or who were in hospital for a relatively brief period compared to asylum admissions.

The first two groups were the focus of the first stage of the process of deinstitutionalisation. In theory, the second two groups would benefit from the establishment of community mental health centres and other changes to the provision of mental health care. Community care represents what now might seem the idealistic belief that the closure of the asylums would represent a hugely progressive shift in the care and treatment of the mentally ill. There are several narratives of community care that are examined in this volume. One of the most powerful is that community care was an inherently progressive idea based on inclusive notions of citizenship. This narrative is based on a view that sees asylums as Gothic sites of seclusion and terror. As Scull (1986) noted, this modern view of the asylum is a betrayal of its origins and would have shocked the founders of these institutions. Figures such as Tuke at the York Retreat established them as progressive and a humanitarian response to suffering. The debates about the causal factors and influence on the development of community care are explored here. What emerges is a complex, messy and often contradictory picture. Progressive idealism, fiscal conservatism and new pharmaceutical developments combined to render the asylum obsolete. The progressive drive for community care was based on the idea that the discredited asylum would be replaced with a range of properly resourced community-based resources to support citizens in acute distress. I think it is clear that this ambitious goal was never achieved. Turner and Columbo (2008) argued risk assessment has replaced an ethic of care as the main focus of service user contact. An understanding of the rise and fall of the asylums, the radical challenge to psychiatry and the subsequent failings of community care is important if we are to appreciate how to build new models of service provision.

The rise of the asylum

One way of understanding the development of community care is to see it as a response to the failings of the asylum regime. The asylum is situated physically apart from the wider community (Pilgrim and Rogers, 2014). This physical distancing, subsequently, became a metaphor for the social and civic isolation of the patients. These institutions were built on sites away from the main centres of population thus physically separating the mad from the rest of the population. Scull (1977) sees the rise of asylums as part of the Victorian response to the problems of urbanisation. In tracing the rise of the asylum, Scull (1977,1986) outlines the way that the institution was linked to and played a role in the new status of psychiatry as a distinct branch of the medical profession. Scull (1986) was particularly critical of Foucault and those who viewed asylums simply as forms of social control. He notes that there was an optimism in this period that contrasts strongly with the end of the asylum period. The new asylums were established to rescue the mad from the kinds of maltreatment and neglect with which they became synonymous. The hospital was a rational, technical response to mental illness.

Michel Foucault is one of the most influential and widely cited writers in the humanities and social sciences. His work and the responses to it have opened new areas of debate. Foucault's work is complex and often appears contradictory. The key themes that he explored include: the nature of power; the development of modern institutions, such as prisons and psychiatric hospitals; and modern modes of social regulation. Foucault argues that these shifts in what he terms 'technologies of power' cannot be necessarily seen as progressive. They reflect changes in the dynamics of societal power. His work on two key institutions of modernity – the asylum and the prison – has at its core a concern with the exercise of power (Foucault, 2003). His work is a challenge to the traditional notion that the development of these institutions can be read as a process of reform. Foucault sees these institutions as new technologies of power. The task is to examine the shifts in social, cultural and political beliefs that underpin these reforms.

Foucault's work is, unlike that of other critics of the asylum regime, historical. He explores the birth of these modern institutions. His influence was and is such that it was taken to be a criticism of contemporary systems (Cummins, 2017). Foucault outlines the way that the focus of punishment and treatment moves from the body of prisoners or patients to their minds. He argues that this is a more pervasive form of social control. In this analysis, power and the power to punish are much more dispersed throughout the social system. It therefore operates on several levels. Foucault terms this ideology of discipline 'savior'. Expressions of this ideology can be found among all groups including those termed deviants and it operates as a mechanism of repression both of the self and others. A subject is created by a series of what he terms 'dividing practices' (Foucault, 1982). These 'dividing practices' are the application of a branch of knowledge such as psychiatry or criminology. The application of such knowledge, for

Foucault creates new groups or cases or in as he puts it 'specifications of individuals'. The implications of being placed in such a category are potentially profound. These include being institutionalised and being denied the rights of citizenship. Foucault argues that the 'Great Confinement' saw the development of institutionalisation as the response to the poor, mad or offenders. In *Discipline and Punish* (2012), Foucault outlines the development of the 'disciplinary gaze'. This is the process by which individuals become cases subject to a system of classification and control. In his writings, Foucault draws attention to the symbolism of the institutions. Bentham's panoptican becomes not just an architectural design but an embodiment of new society, whose institutions form a 'carceral archipelago' for the management of deviant populations, be they criminals or the insane (Foucault, 2003).

It would be a mistake to assume that there were not attempts to respond to the radical perspectives of Foucault and others. The liberal view of the asylum highlights that they represent progress on the previous system. The motives of reformers are fundamentally humanitarian and focusing on the relief of the pain and suffering of their fellow citizens (Jones, 1960). This is an approach that does not see these institutions solely in terms of exercising functions of social control. Individuals such as Tuke, the founder of the York Retreat, are represented as challenging the more hostile views of wider society. By contrast, Foucault (2003) never seems to acknowledge that there is a possibility that some reforms might have been the result of humanitarian concerns. This liberal progressive view of the development of asylums is based on several key premises. It sees mental illness as just that illness and as such a feature of the human condition. Those involved in its treatment and management are motivated by social values to relieve suffering (Ignatieff, 1985). There is, therefore, a key role for the medical profession. This is seen as a logical outcome and allows for the application of rational, morally neutral medical knowledge to the symptoms of mental illness. This creates a narrative of reform involving the improvement of services by the application of new knowledge (Rothman, 2002)

Anti-psychiatry

Anti-psychiatry is a term for a series of critical perspectives on psychiatry that appeared in the 1960s and 1970s. Key thinkers including Goffman (2017), Foucault (2003), Scull (1977), Laing (1959,1967) Fanon (2008) and Szasz (1963,1971) produced a series of highly influential works that questioned the fundamental position of psychiatry. It should be emphasised that this was never a grouping or an intellectual school. They had little if anything in common.

Despite this, it is possible to identify key themes in the work of this diverse group of thinkers that was influential in challenging the dominant model of institutionalised care. I would identify these as follows:

- a fundamental questioning of the exercise of power of the psychiatric profession;
- a questioning of the neutrality of diagnosis;
- a concern with psychiatry's role in the creation and perpetuation of racial and gender stereotypes;
- a belief that institutional care and compulsory treatment were inevitably abusive and dehumanising.

In the broadest terms, these are thinkers of the Left. Szasz is something of an outlier. Szasz is a small government libertarian. He sees mental illness as a way of avoiding individual social responsibility – be that in the area of criminal law or employment. Mental illness in his work is a form of malingering that is indulged by an overgenerous welfare state. His views are neatly summed up in the title of a 1995 paper 'Idleness and lawlessness in the therapeutic state'. It would be a mistake to overlook the differences in other accounts – hence Scull's somewhat sardonic summarising. In critical accounts, there is a sceptical approach which focuses on the social construction of mental illness. This leads to a consideration of broader social factors, such as poverty, racism, misogyny, homophobia and social inequality, rather than a focus on brain chemistry. Following on from this, the social implications of diagnosis and an analysis of the institutions that have been created to manage mental illness are at the heart of anti-psychiatry. For example, while most commentators see the development of the York Retreat as a progressive measure, Foucault (1982) essentially sees it as the exercise of power by other means. He describes the 'moralising sadism' of the York Retreat and its Quaker founders. In Foucault's terms the outcomes for the inmates are the same: exclusion and subjugation. There is a nihilism at the centre of Foucault's thinking. Stone (1982) argued that this leads Foucault to see all relationships in terms of power/subjugation, thus excluding any humanitarian impulse that might underpin to the development of these institutions. It should be acknowledged that in his exchange with Stone, Foucault disputed this interpretation of his work.

Psychiatry and anti-psychiatry

Anti-psychiatry cannot be regarded as a campaigning movement. However, it was clearly influential outside of academic circles. It needs to be considered as a key influence on the development of community care (Cummins, 2017). The key figures remained influential in debates about the nature of mental illness during their lifetimes. Laing set up therapeutic communities; Szasz campaigned against the power of psychiatry as a profession while still practising it. It would be almost impossible to overestimate the influence of Goffmann or Foucault. Both are in the most cited writers in the social sciences (Green, 2016).

Psychiatry, clearly, did not simply accept without challenge the criticisms outlined in the previous paragraph. It is interesting that three of the strongest critics of the discipline were actually psychiatrists – Laing, Szasz and Cooper, who is usually credited with coining the term 'anti-psychiatry'. The response has come from both medicine and the humanities. The strongest arguments are that the main aim of medicine is humanitarian and altruistic: the relief of suffering (Clare, 2012; Wing, 1978) Within these accounts, there is an acceptance that certain practices would now be regarded as abusive or even amount to torture. However, the argument is that this was the state of medical knowledge at the time. The intention was therapeutic within the medical definitions of the time. This is one of the fundamental departures in Foucault's work. In it, it is difficult to find any recognition of the possibility of a humanitarian impulse. I may be guilty here of applying modern notions of therapeutic interventions to the past where they are not applicable.

Alongside what we might term the moral defence of psychiatry – the notion that it is a branch of medicine that is concerned with the relief of suffering – we should also explore other challenges to Foucault. Scull (1991) is very critical of Foucault's use of sources and the conclusions that he reaches arguing they are based on the analysis of a limited range of texts. In addition, Scull (1991) argues that Foucault has used a very specific period in French history to represent the totality of European developments in this field. Sedgwick (1982) has demonstrated that the link Foucault makes between the decline in the treatment of leprosy and the development of psychiatric asylums does not hold. For Foucault, prior to the 'Great Confinement' the mad had essentially been tolerated and allowed to live in society. Sedgwick argues that this portrayal of the mad as the lepers of modern society ignores the fact that the mad had been held in various forms of custody prior to the period Foucault is discussing. In representing asylums as a response to urbanisation, Foucault cannot account for their development in the US at a time when it was an agrarian society (Rothman, 2002). One response to this is to argue that Foucault is not making any such claims. His work is historically specific and seeks to analyse the various factors at play – at that time, in that place. This is counter to an approach that is based on or creates a metanarrative of the rise of the asylums.

For other critics, such as Rothman (2002), Foucault has, in effect, reduced the complex causes of the development of asylums to a class strategy of 'divide and rule'. One impact of this is to simplify the complexity of the founding and management of the asylum regime. For example, it overlooks or does not accept the religious motivations of many founders – Tuke at York being a prime example. Anti-psychiatry chimed with some of the anti-authoritarian developments in the wider culture of the 1960s. This helps to explain the largely positive reception that it received. However, it is also part of its weakness. Scull (2014) demonstrates that all societies grapple with the moral and ethical questions that are generated by societal responses to mental illness. The response clearly involves social control, but we also need to see it as something more than that. There are many aspects to it because mental illness is such a diverse and complex phenomenon. Finally, the focus in Foucault's account is on essentially state responses. This overlooks the other ways that families, wider social attitudes and public sanctions – formal and otherwise –combine to produce social order (Ignatieff, 1985).

Foucault (2003) and Goffman (2017) challenge established notions of progress. They also question the role of psychiatry, viewing it as a disciplinary process. The focus is often on the impact of the asylum regime on the incarcerated. There is a danger of overstating this. For example, the voice of the service user/patient is largely if not totally absent from Goffman (2017). The influence of these writers has led to an explosion in research and literature that explores all aspects of the asylum. The history of the asylum from below is, perhaps, more attractive than a narrative of the struggle of psychiatrists to humanise an inhumane system. However, it is important to examine all aspects of the asylum regime. The fundamental difficulty with these hugely influential accounts is that they are based on a discourse of subordination and domination. In challenging the notion of progress, there seems to be a denial of its possible existence whatsoever. Unfairly in my view, Foucault seems to be held personally responsible by many for the failings of community care. Stone (1982), for example, argues Foucault had a destructive impact on the development of mental health services, arguing the attacks on institutional care led to a collapse in the belief in care itself.

Conclusion

As noted, the progressive proponents of community care saw the abuses of the asylum system as a fundamental human rights issue. Institutionalised forms of treatment were inherently abusive as they denied people the full rights of citizenship and subjected them to inhumane and degrading treatment. For fiscal conservatives, the asylums were part of an increasingly unaffordable welfare state. In later chapters, I explore how the progressive vision of community care disappeared. By 1998, and the arrival of the first New Labour administration, community care had officially 'failed'. One is tempted to respond that it had never really been tried. The sweeping statement that it had failed ignores the fact that there were and are people who would previously been institutionalised, who have not been and are living independently. However, the grander vision of a series of community mental health and crisis centres that would replace the large glooming presence of the asylum has never materialised.

The assumption that there is a binary of the asylum/community and that they are always in opposition is something of an illusion. The idea that all the problems raised by the asylum regime could be solved by a return to the community ignored more fundamental questions about the nature of mental health services. The impulse behind community care was to improve the standards of mental health provision. The overwhelming majority of writers accept that there will be a need for a period of recovery that involves a therapeutic setting of one sort or another. The York Retreat and others like it were just that – a retreat from the pressures of the world. Even a writer as radical as Laing accepted this and set up therapeutic communities as a result. This is not to deny that is that prolonged periods of hospital care can in themselves be damaging and that services need to exist to intervene at an early stage to provide support to those suffering from any form of mental distress. This is a public health model of service provision that ideally develops tiers that will meet individual and community need. Community care from the late 1980s onwards appears as a policy with few vocal supporters. This is partly due to the media coverage of high-profile cases (Cummins, 2010, 2012). One should, perhaps, not be too shocked that the tabloid media, which did so much to contribute to the stigma that users of mental health services face, reported these cases in such a lurid fashion. These reports undermined wider support for the policy. The response has been a call for more coercive legislation, one which ultimately led to the introduction of Community Treatment Orders.

Moon (2000) highlights the geographical paradox at the heart of the development of community care services: the closure of the asylums has not resolved the marginalisation of those experiencing mental health problems. The asylums were distant institutions geographically and metaphorically (Philo 1987; Scull 1989). The notion of community care was based on an inclusive vision. In tracing the history of community care, this volume seeks to examine why that vision never materialised. Far from being a welcoming, supportive environment, communities, particularly in urban areas, have reproduced the worst aspects of the asylum (Wolff, 2005). Those with the most complex needs are often found living in the poorest neighbourhoods, in poor quality residential care homes, on the streets or increasingly in the prison system (Moon, 2000; Singleton et al, 1998). The overall picture is a very bleak one, so bleak in fact that the asylum system appears to have some advantages in that it was, at least, a community. For a variety of reasons – economic, social and political – the community has not proved up to the task of providing humane and effective services for those with the most complex needs.

Mental health services have always struggled to gain an appropriate level of funding – particularly in comparison with other areas of medicine. This is partly a reflection of the stigma attached to the area. The period that is mostly examined in this volume (1983–97) was one that saw a broader restructuring of the welfare state. These pressures meant community care was never properly funded (Scull, 1986). One of the main conclusions of a series of inquiries into failures in community care services (Ritchie, 1994; Blom-Cooper et al, 1995) was that resources were stretched to breaking point. It is interesting to note that these inquiries called for more investment in mental health services but focused on the need for more secure provision. In addition, there were calls for changes in mental health legislation. When examining these issues, it is impossible to separate mental health services from the wider discourses of risk and risk management that came to dominate social work, in particular, as well as other public services (Cummins, 2018a).

The critics of the asylum regime from a human rights perspective were clearly not arguing that they should be replaced by prisons, police custody, homelessness and poor quality bed and breakfast accommodation. The treatment of mental illness is fundamentally a moral issue that involves questions about the rights of the individual and the wider society (Eastman and Starling, 2006). Such questions did not disappear because of the advent of community care. The powers of compulsory admission have remained largely unchanged. The reform of the Mental Health Act (MHA) in 2007 saw the introduction of Community Treatment Orders legislation. This could be taken as the symbolic ending of a policy commitment to community care. These debates are the result of the nature and impact of mental illness. It is only, perhaps, on the more extreme wings of libertarian thought (Szasz 1963, 1971) that there is a total rejection of the therapeutic state having powers to intervene when individuals, because of their mental health, are seen as putting themselves or others at risk in some way. One of the many paradoxes of community care is that the rights of the mentally ill are on a much stronger footing than they have ever been. In the US, challenges to the legal processes of detention were one of the key drivers of deinstitutionalisation (Harcourt, 2005). In the UK, greater legal protections exist that mean people can challenge, for example, employers if they experience discrimination as a result of their mental health problems. In cases of compulsory detention, a new legal framework was introduced to ensure compatibility with the provisions of the HRA (Human Rights Act) of 1998. The 2018 review of the MHA was carried after May identified the parlous state of mental health services as one of the 'grave injustices' that existed in the country. There is wider public discussion and acknowledgement of the impact of mental illness. Stigma and fear remain but the physical segregation in asylums has gone. In addition, psychiatry, mental health social work, nursing and other disciplines have a wider range of interventions to alleviate distress to offer. However, the policies and legislation which will impact on those in greatest need do not reflect these progressive themes. These paradoxes will be explored in the forthcoming chapters.

3

The asylum and the community

Introduction

This chapter will argue that the development of mental health policy was hugely influenced by conceptions of space and place. By the middle of the 20th century the asylum had become, in the public and sociological imagination, a Gothic institution of seclusion and abuse. This is not to suggest that there was no basis for this view. The chapter will explore the development of this representation of the asylum. The final representations of the asylum contrast dramatically with the original ones that saw the new institutions as modern and progressive. Deinstitutionalisation was to present the community in binary opposition to the asylum. Community based services would, almost by reason of their location, lead to the creation of a new form of inclusive mental health provision. This is based on an idealised notion of community. As the pressures on mental health services grew, a range of social policies that were introduced that meant that urban communities, in particular, became exclusionary rather than inclusionary.

Total institutions

Goffman is one of the most influential sociologists of the 20th century. Goffman's work on stigma and the sociology of everyday life – the social practices that we engage in to structure and make sense of day to day social interactions – have left a rich legacy. It is interesting to note that the treatment and management of mental illness was a key area of analysis in his work. This area was representative of other stigma generating processes (Cummins, 2017a). *Asylums* (2017) is Goffman's most important work in this field. It is an ethnographic account of life at the St Elizabeth's Hospital in Washington DC. Goffman carried out his research when there were over 7,000 patients at St Elizabeth's. The study is a landmark in ethnographic research. It also had a key role in the moves to tackle the abusive nature of the regime he described. Goffman's portrait of the asylum was one dominated by essentially anti-therapeutic, dehumanising practices. Goffman's work was part of the drive for reform but also had a key role in shaping the image of the asylum regime.

Before examining *Asylums* (2017), I will briefly outline Goffman's broader theoretical approach to the questions raised by societal responses to mental illness. He examined these in his short essay 'The insanity of place' (Goffman, 1969). Goffman regarded mental illness as a challenge to normal societal rules of behaviour. It represents what he terms a form of 'havoc'. Goffman uses the term to mean that individuals are no longer what he termed self-governing. The usual codes or systems which enable us to make sense of, or manage, our social realities are broken down. An example of this might be the impact of symptoms of bipolar disorder such as disinhibition. For Goffman, society manages havoc in one of two ways: the removal of the individuals from wider society, or the discrediting of them. Goffman outlined what he termed 'gathering' whereby the wider society – families, friends and institutions – attempt to deal with the havoc. As a former mental health social worker, I was involved in many gatherings in the form of Mental Health Act (MHA) assessments. I, my fellow mental health professionals and members of individuals' families viewed Goffman's gatherings as interventions that were seeking to ensure the safety of individuals rather than to discredit them. I also fully accept that my perspective may well be completely at odds with that of the person subject to the MHA assessment process. Alongside this, I accept that these processes include an inevitable element of discrediting and stigmatising the person subject to the assessment.

Goffman used the term 'total institution' to describe asylums. The term was coined by the American sociologist Everett Hughes who taught at the University of Chicago when Goffman was a postgraduate student. A total institution is one where the basic modern social arrangements whereby individuals sleep, play and work 'in different places, with different co-participants, under different authorities, and without an overall rational plan' (Goffman, 2017: 5–6) are broken down. Those living in total institutions are separated from the wider society. Barracks, monasteries, psychiatric hospitals, prisons and residential and nursing homes could all be regarded as total institutions or have features of total institutions. A total institution is not necessarily based on compulsory admission. This is important: people make a positive choice to enter a monastery. Not all admissions to psychiatric hospital are compulsory but the nature of the choice made is open to debate. Not all total institutions are based on a desire to exclude; they may be the result of a positive decision to reject aspects of modern society. The barriers that exist between three spheres of modern life

– sleep, play and work – are broken down or disappear completely. The result is that residents/patients/inmates conduct all aspects of their lives in the same restricted physical and psychological environment. In Goffman's psychiatric model, this environment is also a controlled one, dominated by a staff group that has power over the way that all aspects of the institution are organised and function. The regime is imposed by a system of explicit formal rules but also a second system of informal ones, overseen and imposed by the staff group. The aim of the regime is to control the havoc that led to the inmate/patient admission so that they can re-enter mainstream society.

In St Elizabeth's, Goffman (2017) noted that the ward system was not based totally on clinical need. It had a clear disciplinary function. The ward system is an example of the way that staff exercise authority and control. For Goffman, the system was a purely behaviourist one. Behaviourism was a dominant approach in psychiatric institutions in this period. Those patients who cooperated were sent to the 'best wards'. The most uncooperative patients were sent to the wards where the conditions were poorest. The total institution followed a clear system of rewards for good behaviour and punishment for acts seen as transgression. The rewards included improved conditions, but also access to TV and radio or cups of coffee. One of the sharpest insights that Goffman (2017) provides is into the way that individuals respond to the strictures and demands of the total institution. He recognises that within the limitations of the asylum regime, individuals attempt to – and in fact are driven to – maintain their identity. This inevitably involves some transgression of the asylum rules. Goffman highlights the way that the all-pervasive nature of the asylum regime means that behaviour in one area of a person's life is brought into another, providing evidence that the 'spoiled identity' assigned to them is a valid one. Rosenhan (1975) made a similar point when he argued that one of the most power aspects of diagnosis was that it became a prism through which all behaviour is examined and explained.

Asylums (Goffman, 2017) is, or should be, on the reading list for every mental health module on social work, sociology and social policy courses. The strength of the work is that it examines how response to mental illness becomes a form of social control. Scull (1986) also highlights this as the fundamental weakness of Goffman's analysis. It does not allow for any therapeutic motivations. The cultural influence of *Asylums* can be seen in a number of representations of mental illness – most notably in Ken Kesey's (1962) novel *One Flew over the Cuckoo's Nest* (and Milos Forman's 1975 multi Oscar winning film adaptation of the book). The character of McMurphy and Jack Nicholson's portrayal of him in the film became iconic representations of the main themes of the anti-psychiatry movement (Cummins, 2017b). The character – serving a prison sentence for statutory rape – is presented as a rebel against the abuses of the regimes but also the wider conformity of post war US consumer society. In his analysis, Goffman excluded the possibility that the asylum could be viewed as an attempt to respond to human suffering. This is clearly not an attempt to defend abusive practices. It is to suggest that *Asylums* fails to place these institutions in a clear historical context. There is a streak of nihilism that runs through his work that is echoed in Foucault.

The current view of the asylum is largely dominated by its representation as a Gothic institution. Tuan (1979) described them as key markers in 'landscapes of fear'. Ironically, many of the design features, outlined in the next section, that were seen as therapeutic at the time add to this image. In 1954 there were still 154,000 patients in British mental hospitals. The criticisms of these institutions grew in the 1950s and 1960s. Barton (1959) identified the negative effects that institutionalisation could have on patients, comparing the behaviour of patients on long-stay wards to similar behaviour that he had seen of prisoners in concentration camps. Scott (1973) argued that the hospital itself made individuals passive. This meant that they would be unable to cope with life outside the institution. This followed earlier work by Wing (1962), which had shown how the process of social withdrawal developed among long-stay patients. Overall the picture is one of a physically, socially and culturally isolated institutions cut off from the main stream of health care and the wider society. Martin (1985) described the systemic faults in the institutional provision as the 'corruption of care'. As discussed in Chapter 3, scandals about the abuse of patients and subsequent public exposure of them became one of the powerful drivers of moves to reform.

Asylum

The term asylum originally meant a place of refuge, safety and protection. This is reflected in its usage in modern international law. Asylum is the protection granted by one state to citizens who have fled another state because of political oppression or fear of persecution. It is the right of a state to grant asylum – it can be refused. In more recent times, asylum seeker has been consistently used in the tabloid press as a term of abuse (Tyler, 2013). Scull (1986) notes that the modern treatment and management of mental illness involved an expansion of state institutions. These institutions were accompanied by the rise of specialists – *alienists*, the forerunner of the modern psychiatrist – who were able apply their specialist knowledge and skills to the identification, assessment and subsequent treatment of groups or individuals.

The publicly funded asylum did not emerge in England until the 19th century. Prior to this period, there was a system of private madhouses where the wealthy were able to place disturbed relatives. These madhouses were often small and not subject to regulation. Abuse was common and a series of scandals led to a Parliamentary Inquiry and eventually An Act for Regulating Private Madhouses (1774). There were a series of scandals and debates about the treatment of the mentally ill in this period. William Tuke opened the York Retreat in 1796. The funds for the Retreat were raised by the local Quaker community in response to the appalling treatment of Hannah Mills, who died in the York Lunatic Asylum. The system of moral treatment that Tuke helped to develop was based in Quaker informed principles of treating individuals with respect and dignity. The 1828 County Asylums Act saw the establishment of a more formal admissions process but also an inspection regime that provided annual reports to Parliament. In 1845, the Lunatic Asylums Act placed a duty on counties to establish a pauper asylum. This led to a huge expansion in the number of asylums that became such important features of the physical and cultural landscape.

This illustrates that there was a clear humanitarian impulse in the development of the asylum system (Scull, 1986). The later crisis in asylums obscures or marginalises this (Cummins, 2017a). The geographical position and architecture of the asylums were cited by its 20th century critics as evidence of an ideology that sought to banish or exclude the mentally ill and other undesirables from the wider society (Foucault, 2003; Goffman, 2017). This was not the case at the time. Many asylums such as the one in York were called Retreats for the very specific reason that they were just that – a place to escape the pressures of the modern world. One of Scull's (1986) main criticisms of Goffman (2017) is that he fails to acknowledge that this at any point. As outlined, Goffman (2017) saw the institution as creating the difficulties that the patients face. There is hardly any consideration of the issues that led to their admission. This is, of course, not to deny that abuses took place or that the impact of admission. It is simply to acknowledge the complexity of these processes.

The asylum was planned for a very specific purpose. It is a representation of an ideological response to the problem of madness (Franklin, 2002). The same is equally true of the modern notions of community, which form the basis of community care. The asylums built following the 1845 County Asylum Act were often designed by famous architects such as Sir George Gilbert Scott, a leading figure in the Victorian Revival. In his early career, he designed hundreds of workhouses. His most famous designs include the Albert Memorial and the main building of the University of Glasgow. Charles Fowler, who designed Covent Garden Market, was responsible for an asylum in Devon. The asylums were thus important civic statements. The great architect critic Sir Nikolaus Pevsner praised a number of asylum designs for the scope and ambition of their design. The Victorian Society and other conservation groups have campaigned for the listing of asylums because of their architectural heritage.

The asylums of the Victorian period were located outside of urban settings. This distance from the urban environment and the large grounds that often surrounded them was a key feature of moral treatment. Fresh air and other aspects of the rural idyll were seen as having recuperative properties. The asylums were built on rural slightly elevated sites to avoid the dangers of miasma – foul smelling vapours that were the result of poor sanitation. Until the development of germ theory, it was believed that miasma spread disease (Franklin, 2002). The early asylums were small with a couple of hundred patients. The 1845 Act led to the building of bigger institutions. The other important design features included separate wards for men and women as well as different wards for patients suffering from different conditions. Wards were built facing south with access to a court where patients were able to experience fresh air and sunshine – key elements of the therapy (Franklin, 2002). The corridor plan of these asylums was based on the sanitary principles proposed by Florence Nightingale. The asylum designs often included a house for the medical superintendent, workshops, recreation hall, a ballroom, a farm, a brewery, a chapel and a mortuary. The effect was the creation of a small self-contained community.

In examining a range of perspectives on the development of asylums, it is important not to paint an unrealistic picture or ignore the abuses that occurred or the damage that was done to individuals. Parr et al (2003) in their discussion of the Craig Dunain Hospital near Inverness show that the patients' narratives of the institution are much more complex and contradictory than is sometimes allowed for. The authors note that the institution had a negative reputation with outside observers. However, the memories of the staff and patients were much more nuanced and complex. The former patients highlighted the lack of personal space and the accompanying indignities. For example, there was no real privacy so patients received injections or had consultations with their doctors in what amounted to public spaces on the ward. At the same time, the former patients spoke about the friendships that they had developed. The grounds of the asylum were particularly fondly remembered as a place where patients were able to enjoy a measure of personal freedom – smoke cigarettes, have intimate relationships and so on. The asylum in this approach is viewed as a much more complex and ambiguous set of social and physical relationships than is allowed for Goffman's total institution narrative. As one former resident put it 'That awful place was home' (Parr, 2003). In Parr et al's (2003) study the former patients of Craig Dunain are very critical of the new functionalist mental health facility that replaced it – describing it as soulless.

The asylum may have physically disappeared from the landscape, but it remains a potent cultural reference point. There are any number of computer games and apps such as 'Adventure Escape: Asylum' which are based on the Gothic image of the asylum. In this game, for example, the marketing plays to a number of tropes that occur across the horror genre:

> Anna wakes up one day in an asylum with hazy memories of her past. Soon, it's clear that something has gone very, very wrong at the Byers Institute. In fact, there is a killer on the loose. (Google Play, no date)

In addition, there are several modern novels that explore the experience of asylums. These include Lehane's (2003) tribute to B movies and pulp fiction *Shutter Island*, where a detective is called to a hospital for the criminally insane to investigate the disappearance of a patient. In Maggie O'Farrell's (2006) Costa award winning novel *The Vanishing Act of Esme Lennox,* the title character has spent her adult life in an Edinburgh asylum. The novel explores the reasons why her family sought to have her institutionalised.

The process of deinstitutionalisation created the question: what should be done with the sites of the asylums? One of the ironies was that the geographical position of the asylum meant that they were now prime sites for development. Cummins (2018) notes that the site of the former asylum in Gorizia that was closed as part of Basaglia's reforms of the Italian system became a public park. In the UK of the 1980s and 1990s, the focus was much more on private provision – housing and shopping developments. The heritage status of some sites led to the retention of the buildings as part of prestige developments (Chaplin and Peters, 2003), with the substantial grounds being a bonus. These luxury housing developments use a language of sanctuary that has echoes of the asylum narrative. The development is a private space that offers an escape from the pressures of the city but convenient access to it. This is, of course, required as the buyers will need to work in lucratively paid jobs to afford such an exclusive property. Chaplin and Peters (2003) note that the advertising for such developments uses terms such as 'seclusion' that had generally negative overtones when the space was an asylum. The authors found that there were few explicit references to the fact that these developments were on the sites of former asylums. The stigma attached to the asylum lingers on, even after the institution itself has physically disappeared. However, as Chaplin and Peters conclude, 'paradoxically, asylum can now be bought in an ideal self-contained community, with security to keep society out' (Chaplin and Peters, 2003: 228).

Leary (2011) outlines what he calls 'ruin pornography', by this he means the stylish and artistic photographs and media representations of once great industrial cities. He terms this trend Detroitism, as the city has gone from being a metonym for post war growth to one for deindustrialisation. As he points out, it is possible to buy art house coffee table books of ruined and neglected buildings that were once the heartbeat of US post war industrial economic boom. What these photographs cannot capture is the dynamism of a booming economy or what that meant for working class people. The stylised photographs and images obviously cannot capture the reality of these areas as working environments – the heat, the noise and the physical effort required to keep up with industrial processes are all missing. In a rather similar vein, there is a thriving interest in neglected and abandoned asylums. These photographs are used, in a similar way, to capture the essence of the former institutions. These haunting photographs of abandoned wards, strange equipment used in treatments and images of neglected patients all add to the Gothic reputation of the asylum. 'Asylumism' thus acts as a metonym for the management and treatment of mental illness before the advent of community care. In doing so, it collapses the end of the asylum as an institution into its whole history.

Van der Velde (2016) published *Abandoned Asylums* – a series of photographs that promises readers 'an unrestricted visual journey inside America's abandoned state hospitals, asylums and psychiatric facilities, the institutions where countless stories and personal dramas played out behind locked doors and out of public sight'. It also promises images of hospitals that treated the famous and infamous, including Marilyn Monroe and Charles Manson. The abandoned and decaying institutions act as magnets for so-called 'urban explorers', such as Keïtaï, who enter abandoned sites and post photographs of what they find. Alongside a series of photographs, the following is an entry from Keïtaï's blog about a visit to the former West Park Asylum in Epsom Surrey.

> We were able to see more of the place; the padded cell, the main hall, the post office and the children's creche. The padded cell was our main goal like many others who venture there. It was smaller then [sic] I expected and harder too. (Keïtaï, 2011)

This is not the only approach to the complex history of the asylum. For example, 'The lives they left behind: Suitcases from a state hospital attic' (Community Consortium, 2015) is an exhibition based on a suitcases found in an abandoned building when the Willard Psychiatric Center in New York's Finger Lakes closed in 1995. The exhibition paints a complex portrait of the individual lives of the patients before they entered the asylum. This approach forces the reader to ask fundamental questions such as 'why were these individuals admitted to the institution, how were they treated and why were patients for such long periods?' Raymond Depardon produced a series of superb photographs of the Gorizia asylum where Basaglia (Foot, 2015) enacted his reforms. These photographs document the need for the reform, as Depardon in discussing how he came to take the photographs states:

> I often went back to the old hospital in Trieste, the place called the 'manicomio', the 'lunatic asylum'. One day, I followed this group coming out of the canteen. What was it about the patients that struck me: the way they looked, the clothes they wore, the way they walked? I was drawn to them. I found myself in a very old 'reparto;' the door of the ward closed behind me, there wasn't a nurse in sight. With the noise and the decrepitude of the place, I confess that for a moment I took fright. I started taking photographs, very quietly. (Raymond Depardon, quoted in Howard, 2018)

The development of mental health policy is a history of space and place, seclusion and exclusion. In examining this history, it is vital to consider the symbolic value that is placed on particular spaces and places. Bedlam comes to be representative of institutionalised care. In the US, conscientious objectors in the Second World War were sent to work as hospital orderlies in asylums. Parsons (2018) highlights that these individuals were appalled by what they saw and became committed to reform. This initially involved fighting racial segregation. Conscientious objectors working at the Philadelphia State Hospital at Byberry took their concerns to two journalists Alfred Deutsch and Albert Maisel. This resulted, in 1946, in the publication of an expose in *Life* magazine, which reached millions of US citizens – the modern equivalent of a prime time documentary or viral video. The expose compared the hospital to prisons. The article also included a photograph, entitled *Despair*, of an emaciated, naked patient (Parsons, 2018). For readers, who the previous year had seen newsreels of the liberation of Belsen, the link was an obvious one. Later, in 1960s Italy, Basaglia, who was heavily influenced by the work of the Holocaust survivor Primo Levy, made a similar link between the camp and the asylum (Foot, 2015). This was a link that Levy did not think stood up to scrutiny (Cummins, 2018).

The French historian Pierre Nora considers public memory and sites of commemoration, He noted that there is a 'rapid slippage of the present into a historical past that is gone for good' (Nora, 1989: 7). He argued that we respond to this by focusing on memories of physical spaces. Thus, the modern world becomes obsessed with a socially constructed version of history that can replace previous collective memories (Nora, 1989). He coined the term *lieux de mémoire* for sites of remembrance. Nora (1989) sees memory and history as being in opposition with each other. He states: 'History's goal and ambition is not to exact but to annihilate what has in reality taken place' (Nora, 1989: 9). He uses the battlefields of Verdun. The site has become a national monument to the Fallen. In creating the memorials, the horror and carnage has been removed. In its place, there is a grandeur and solemnity totally at odds with the battle that the site commemorates. One possible way to approach asylums is to see them as *lieux de mémoire* where the memories are still contested.

Community

As previously outlined, the asylum was an institution set apart both physically and psychology from the wider society. This exclusion also reflected the way that psychiatry was a discipline apart from others in medicine. One of the drivers of community care was to tackle this social isolation of the psychiatric patient. There was an implicit assumption that the ills of institutionalisation would be overcome by community based services. Community is one of Raymond Williams' *Keywords* (2014). *Keywords* (Williams, 2014) is an exploration of the changing meanings of the words and terms that are used in discussions of culture and cultural ideas. It consists of 110 short essays on terms including bourgeois, culture and hegemony. He published a revised version in 1983, and added 21 new words.

In 2018, MacCabe and Yanacek edited a new collection – *Keywords for Today*. Community is one of their keywords. Williams had suggested that community is a word that is never used in a negative fashion. They do not consider its use in the phrase community care, which clearly developed negative connotations, in a very relatively short period in the late 1980s and early 1990s. Community is long established in the English language. It originally meant the common people as opposed to those of rank, the people of a local area or the quality of holding something in common (MacCabe and Yanacek, 2018). The authors note that, as society became more complex, community was the word used for alternative approaches to group living, for example, a religious community. This use made its way into the history of mental health – for example Laing's establishment of therapeutic communities (Cummins, 2017a). These communities were self-contained and in a sense self-governing. They were attempts to live an alternative, healthier life. The use of community has spread. It is used in a broader political sense – for example the emergence of the term gay community in the 1980s – to represent a grouping of individuals with a shared social identity or shared political and cultural interests. It should be noted that this use of the term is fraught with difficulties. It assumes that there is a commonality of interests which might not necessarily be the case. The notion of community politics is used to denote a more informal, localised approach to campaigning. This is presented as a purer form of political activity. Here community stands in opposition or contrast to the tainted world of machine politics. In one of those ironies of usage, in recent times, there has been the emergence of 'gated communities' – as previously noted, a number on the site of former asylums. The use of community plays to notion of inclusion and a nostalgic vision of what life used to be while they are gated to ensure that unwanted elements are kept out.

Community, then, is a term that carries within it elements of nostalgia but also positive notions of making better social connections between individuals and groups. There remains a sense of flexibility in the use of the term community. It can be used as a cipher for a range of values. In the political and policy sphere, it is used as a marker to claim that there is something of an ethical core to proposals. For Bauman (2001) community acts as a counter to a more individualised present or Rose's (1996) 'death of the social'. Thus, community is presented as the solution to a whole range of social and other problems. However, we cannot find the mechanisms that will help to recreate it (Bauman, 2001). These trends seem to have become more entrenched since the development of social media. Social media creates communities of a different sort to the organic forms that are the basis of these debates.

Arendt (1959) argues that some form of commonality is central to our physical survival. Individualism and autonomy are core values of our increasingly dislocated community. However, there are contradictions here as we cannot survive without care from others – as infants but also at other times in our lives (Fineman, 2004). The notion of community is a powerful one. In his analysis of nationalism, Anderson (2006) argued that a nation is 'an imagined political community' – this is true of all nations. Politicians and elites can make calls based on the idea that though citizens will never meet most of the members of the imagined community, they share interests or an identity. There are periods where this is most keenly felt, for example, major events such as the Olympic Games. This notion of an imagined community can also be applied at a more regional or micro level. Community is an elusive ideal – it is constructed from memory. An idea that is projected into both the past – as it never existed in the way that it is remembered – and the future where it can never exist in the way that it is imagined.

The multiplicity of meanings attached to community allow it to be used with little analytical work (Crow and Allan, 1995). In the late 1970s and early 1980s, as policies of deindustrialisation began to take effect, there was an increasing interest in the notion of community. Community was seen as providing a bulwark against the impact of New Right economic and social policies. Even though many on the Left were attracted to these notions, the use of the term across the political spectrum meant that it was problematic. In particular, the term seems to imply some sense of greater localised, democratic involvement in decision making, but this was often not the case. Policies were often constructed and shaped by the needs of the wider state. The result was that the responsibility for hugely significant social problems was localised limiting the role of state actors and policies in their creation. Brown (2015) notes the way that neoliberal politics pushes the nexus of social problems and their solutions further and further away from the site of their creation. Calls to communities are part of this process. Issues such as class and inequality become marginalised. The language of community is a potentially powerful depoliticising force.

The main expansion of the policy of community care was, somewhat ironically, undertaken by a government whose leader, Thatcher, famously declared that there was no such thing as society. Hall (1979) was one of the first to identify the implications of the shifting political and economic trends of the 1970s. In his seminal essay 'The Great Moving Right Show', Hall (1979) saw that the mixture of economic liberalism and social conservativism that Thatcher represented was a new and influential political force. The essay was published in January 1979 before Thatcher's election victory in May of that year. The post war social democratic settlement was unravelling at that point – most clearly in the winter of discontent (Lopez, 2014). Thatcherism was able to pose as representative of the interests 'ordinary' British citizen against the vested interests of the social democratic welfare state – radical trade unions, teachers and social workers, and so on.

These processes also entail the *Othering* of groups such as BAME communities, the poor, welfare claimants and offenders. Hall was right in his view that Thatcherism marked a break from the post war consensus. Thatcher developed a political image that was the antithesis of consensus, attacking what she saw as the nation's enemies within and without. Thatcher's uses of the symbols of Nation and Empire are excellent examples of Anderson's (2006) 'imagined community' as well as the fact these communities are inevitably exclusionary.

In the city: geographies of exclusion

Members of the Chicago school were the first to develop a spatial theorisation of the city (Soja,1996). Spatial factors play a key role in the creation and maintenance of social and community relationships (Simmel, 2004). The city represents modernity, progress (Park, 1967) and creativity but also a sense of dislocation and danger. At the same time establishes social order (Tonnies, 1955). Any analysis of the deregulated, gentrified city created by modern forms of capitalism has to consider Davis' (1998) *City of Quartz*. Davis' (1998) study of Los Angeles (LA) focuses on the way that urban spaces are sorted and segregated. Urban spaces are the key battle ground where capital establishes and maintains its dominance. Public space is essentially privatised. The poor are excluded so that the middle classes and elites can take advantage of the new leisure culture of city centres. Davis (1998: 224) argues 'Police battle the criminalised poor for valorized spaces'. Value comes from the fact that these are spaces dedicated to consumption and recreation. They therefore need to be protected. The subtitle of *City of Quartz* is 'excavating the future'. The LA model of development and regeneration is one that has been followed across late capitalist societies.

Neoliberal forms of governance saw huge changes to the management of urban environments. This shift was based on a whole series of financial policies, such as free trade zones, deregulation and changes to planning law, that has been characterised as a process of 'creative destruction' (Brenner and Theodore, 2002). Alongside these financial policies a set of social policies including zero tolerance initiatives, clampdowns on anti-social behaviour and increased use of CCTV have attempted to manage the city centres and make them attractive to capital and consumers (Harvey, 1990). In these new urban environments, public space is more limited and other environments, for example shopping malls, are subject to greater forms of surveillance or private policing. These environments are replicated across cities so that they become predictable and somewhat sanitised (Sibley, 1995). Sibley (1995) argues that an integral part of these new developments is 'boundary erection'. These boundaries are physical but also economic and psychological. They are based on conceptions of abjection and hostility. The new boundaries of the modern urban environment are increasingly moral ones (Sibley, 1995: 39–43) The exclusions are based on factors that include class, race and disability. The ultimate division is, perhaps, between consumers and the ultimate deviant in neoliberalism – the non-consumer. In these processes, the value of property is seen as higher than the value of people (Sibley, 1995). If asylums can be viewed as rural, then community care is a policy most closely associated with urban environments. Wacquant (2008) sees the city as a location or means of sorting populations into desirable/ undesirable. This is done on the basis of class and race. However, mental health status also became a factor in these processes (Moon, 2000; Cummins, 2010a).

The period of community care coincided with the initial stages of what came to be termed neoliberalism. These policies led to increased inequality, which has produced social and economic segregation (Savage, 2015). These developments have social, psychological and economic impacts (Wilkinson and Pickett, 2010). There are huge differences between the physical and mental health of the richest and poorest in society. The early development of these increasing divisions can be traced back to the 1980s. These differences are starkest in the most unequal societies. More equal societies with progressive welfare and health systems mitigate these potentially adverse outcomes (Marmot, 2015). There was a brief period under the first New Labour government where increased investment in social welfare halted some of these developments. However, they have been intensified during the austerity since 2010 (Cummins, 2018). In many ways, the progressive arguments for community care in the mental health sector assumed continued broader investment in social welfare provisions. There was an implicit view that a shift from spending money on institutionalised psychiatry to community mental health services would not only take place but also lead to better outcomes for service users.

From the late 1990s onwards, in the UK and across Europe, there has been an ongoing moral panic (Cohen, 2011) about the 'ghettoisation' of socially deprived urban areas. The term ghetto – in modern usage – suggests an area of poor housing, poverty, substance misuse problems, high crime and gang violence. It also has racist overtones.

More recently in the UK, governments of all political persuasions have been concerned with the issue of 'sink' estates. Slater (2018) demonstrates that the term 'sink estate', which is often presented as an academic or sociological term, was invented by journalists. Its use was then extended by free market think tanks before becoming a form of policy doxa. It was used as a shorthand for areas that allegedly create a range of social problems such as poverty, worklessness and welfare dependency. Slater (2009) argues that the ghetto is a social and psychological space with its boundaries created by ethnicity. Although these spaces were originally the result of discrimination, they also generate forms of community organisation.

Wacquant (2008a, 2008b, 2009a, 2009b) suggests that modern, urban, spatially concentrated forms of poverty have made it more difficult to sustain social and community institutions. Fordism had been associated with a range of previously strong civic institutions, ranging from political to social and from trade unions to sports and youth clubs. Changing patterns of employment and the increase in precarity have been a key factor here. It is very important to note that Wacquant is not suggesting that such social systems do not exist. For example, his *Body and Soul* (2000) examines the experience of young black men who use a gym in Chicago and considers the function of these informal structures in some detail. In a similar vein, McKenzie's (2015) portrait of life on a Nottingham estate – *Getting By* – focuses not only on the economic and social pressures facing the residents but also the ways in which they overcome them.

Wacquant (2007) terms this 'territorial stigmatization' – the processes whereby areas are characterised by:

> … forms of poverty that are neither residual, nor cyclical or transitional, but inscribed in the future of contemporary societies insofar as they are fed by the ongoing fragmentation of the wage labour relationship, the functional disconnection

> of dispossessed neighbourhoods from the national and global economies, and the reconfiguration of the welfare state in the polarizing city. (Wacquant, 2007: 66–7)

Media representations of community care as a failing policy focused on either the neglect of patients or an increased risk to the public. The longer the policy was in the public eye, the more the media focus was on the alleged increased risk that former psychiatric patients posed to their fellow citizens. There is a similar arc here to the asylum narratives outlined earlier. The failings of the policy in its later iterations acts as a prism through which the whole prism is viewed. This obscures not only positive aspects of earlier periods but also means that the narratives of those who might have spent their lives in institutions but did not are never examined or are lost. By 1984, there were 71,000 inpatients, roughly half the number when Powell made his Water Tower speech in 1961. Leff and Triemann (2000) argue that the first wave of community care was largely seen as a positive move. This period saw the resettlement of long-stay patients. These patients were, on the whole, better supported by mental health services. One key aspect of this was the fact that resettlement often involved the use of specific funding for that purpose. Later, community care services had to compete with others for access to increasingly squeezed funds.

As with deinstitutionalisation in the US, community care rather rapidly became associated with street homelessness or people living in very poor accommodation. Scull (1986), in criticising the impact of deinstitutionalisation, identifies what he terms a modern trade in lunacy. He notes that the irony of a policy developed to deal with the abuses of the asylum regime leading to concerns about vulnerable people being exploited by unscrupulous private landlords. Similar concerns in the early 19th century had been a driving force in the establishment of the original asylums. In 1976, John Pilger, then a campaigning journalist for the *Daily Mirror*, wrote an expose of the way that psychiatric patients were being discharged to bed and breakfast (B&B) accommodation with no support or follow up. Pilger report is based in Birmingham, which he describes as a 'city of lost souls'. The article reports that former patients are living in crowded, often insanitary conditions. They are often not allowed in the accommodation during the day so spend their time wandering about the city centre as there is little in the way of constructive activity. The social workers that Pilger interviewed for the article suggest that Birmingham, possibly because of its size and the number of B&Bs acts as something of a magnet. They give accounts of psychiatric institutions outside of the city discharging patients with a one-way ticket to Birmingham. When reading the Ritchie Inquiry (Ritchie et al, 1994) and its account of Christopher Clunis's contact with mental health services, which took place 15 years after Pilger's article, one is struck by how often Clunis is living in homeless accommodation – a clearly totally unsuitable environment and one that could not possibly hope to meet his needs.

The asylum was thus not replaced by a well-resourced system of community mental centres, crisis accommodation, supported and independent living schemes and employment, which would enable people with mental health problems to complete the journey from 'patient to citizen' (Sayce, 2000) As the asylum closed, a fragmented, dislocated informal network of bedsits, housing projects, day centres or, increasingly, prisons and the criminal justice system replaced it (Moon, 2000; and Wolff, 2005). For many, as Parr et al (2003) demonstrated the friendship and communal living aspects that existed in asylums were lost. Knowles (2000) in her study of the way that former patients negotiated the public spaces, shopping malls and urban environment of Montreal shows that rather becoming integrated into the wider community, this group was isolated and shunned in similar ways to asylum patients. A series of powerful black and white photographs captures the ways that the 'mad' exist alongside but are ignored by the wider society. Knowles (2000) highlights the ways in which the responsibility for the care of the 'mad' has moved from public to private institutions. She goes on to suggest that the restructuring of mental health services acted as a model for other 'problematic populations'. As Cross (2010) suggests, pre-existing social representations of the 'other' are very powerful in their ability to create a new identity for social categories. In this case, the representation of the mad from the asylum era has followed those people into the community. The homeless mentally ill (black) man became a TV and film drama cliché of gritty urban realism. The representation has changed – the mad are not now dishevelled creatures chained to walls – they are the homeless of the modern city living on the streets with all their belongings in shopping carts. Their presence on the margins is accepted as a feature of modern urban life. In his discussion of asylum seekers, Bauman (2007) argues that in a world of 'imagined communities' they are the 'unimaginable'. Similar processes can be identified here; the mad became one of the constituents of what Bauman termed 'internally excluded'. The media debates about community care led not to calls for investment in community mental health services but changes to legislation and a demand for the return of institutionalised care (Cummins, 2010b).

Conclusion

Mental health and responses to it take place within specific locations – temporal and spatial. The geographical locus of treatment provides an insight into the theoretical underpinnings of treatment but also wider social attitudes. Two idealised notions or representations of the asylum and the community came to play a dominant role in broader understandings of mental health policy. The asylum/community binary contains within it a series of other binaries: past/future; rural/urban; inclusion/exclusion; abuse/dignity; institutionalisation/independence; tradition/modernity; and deterioration/progress. The development of asylums involved the institutionalisation of populations who were regarded in some way as deviant (Castel, 1988, 1989). Asylums were located on the outskirts of cities or in rural settings, partly for therapeutic reasons but also as acts of exclusion. The asylum dominated the landscape in a physical but also a metaphorical sense. The closure of the asylums represented not just the transfer of the location of services but a switch in the modality of service provision (Joseph and Kearns, 1996). The seclusion of the asylum setting and their architecture ironically made them attractive to property developers in the 1980s. Those sites that were abandoned became part of the Gothic myth of the asylum.

Community care was seen as an antithesis to the dehumanising regime of the total institution that Goffman (2014) and others outlined. Community was used in a very problematic way that overlooked some of the philosophical difficulties with the concept. The community was assumed to be an entity rather than an abstraction but also a welcoming one. This proved to be naive, perhaps even wildly optimistic. As community care was being introduced, a series of economic and social policies placed tremendous pressure on the poorest urban communities. The asylum disappeared and its place was a rather hidden world of B&Bs and often poor supported housing projects or homelessness. These moves were at odds with a narrative of independence and civic rights that was to be found in policy documents. Moon (2000: 241) argues that the 'concealed others' of the asylum regime were replaced with the 'visible others' of the new system. The asylum was a site of social hygiene. Community care became associated with the 'street' as a public space of potential danger. These concerns were increased by the series of homicides that are examined in Chapter 3. It led to calls for more the provision of more secure psychiatric beds.

Young (1999) discussed what he termed the 'narrative of modernity'. He saw the Fordist regime of production as leading to a stable pattern of employment supported by a universalist welfare regime. These systems helped to generate a series of social and community bounds. The moves from asylum to community should be viewed as part of wider shifts in society. The asylum came to be seen as an abusive system that denied citizens with mental health problems fundamental rights. The inclusive nature of the Fordist regime was illusory – inclusion for some means exclusion and marginalisation for others (Foucault, 2003). The excluded groups such as women, the poor, people from minority communities and the mentally ill were seen as 'other' – not full citizens in both the legal and moral sense (Nye 2003; Yar and Penna, 2004) The historical narrative of modernity includes an emphasis on the development of individualism and the progressive implementation of Enlightenment ideals. This view was challenged from the 1960s by a number of social movements which included mental health service user groups. Wider democratic developments obscured the treatment and continued exclusion from civil society of marginalised groups (O'Brien and Penna, 1998).

The policy of community care became a domestic policy crisis for the beleaguered Major government (Cummins, 2010a). One of the key ways in which the modern state claims legitimacy is by ensuring public and individual safety. Thus governments must respond to a series of threats such as a possible terrorist attack. These threats are increasingly internal or domestic ones. The 'madman' of tabloid legend became one of these perceived threats to the legitimacy of the 'personal security state'. The option of building new asylums was never seriously considered. This would have required a huge fiscal commitment from the state. A new much looser network of private mental health care provision developed. This was largely hidden from the wider society. Local people might be aware of a small supported housing project but these were usually terraced houses rather than purpose built accommodation. It is a sad reality that the abuse, neglect and marginalisation that took place under the old regime did not end when the asylum gates were closed.

4

Inquiries

Introduction

This chapter will explore a number of mental health inquiries that took place in the early and mid-1990s. It will argue that the media reporting – particularly that in tabloid newspapers – had a key role in undermining support for the progressive elements of community care. This is not to diminish the nature of some of the cases that led to the inquiries. It is, rather, to consider the way that this media reporting helped to construct a discourse around risk and mental health. This reporting played on a series of long standing, often racialised tropes about the nature of mental illness. One of the most important of these was the notion that there is a clear, identifiable and causal link between mental illness and violence. These are complex issues. However, complexity was drowned out by the dominant narrative that the community faced new dangers in the form of 'psychokillers'. Alongside this, a theme in the reporting of such cases was that liberal mental health professionals were refusing to use their powers to intervene.

Before exploring the role of mental health inquiries in the late 1980s and 1990s, it is important to place inquiries in the broader policy and organisational context of New Public Management (NPM). NPM seeks to bring the so-called disciplines of the market to the public sector. According to Pollitt and Bouckaert (2004), NPM was an attempt to introduce some elements of the market, such as competition, to public services. This is part of a shift that saw the marketisation of the state (Hutton, 1996). Health and welfare services have seen huge changes in the funding and delivery of services since the early 1980s. These have included not only the sale of state assets but also the contracting out of services – for example catering, cleaning and other support services – to private companies. Skelcher (2000) outlined three modern models of the state: the overloaded state of the 1960s/1970s; the hollowed-out state of the 1980s/early 1990s; and the congested state of the late 1990s. There is something of a contradiction here as neoliberalism seeks to limit the role of the state to a 'night watchman role' but the role of the state has expanded. This is the case in the area of penal policy (Cummins, 2018) but also in other areas. The demands of late modern capitalism meant that a role was required for the state. For example, all advanced economies require an increasingly well-educated workforce. These demands will not be met by private institutions.

The inquiries that are the focus of this chapter took place in the period that Skelcher (2000) argued saw the 'hollowing out' of the state. This term covers the process where new arrangements for the audit and governance of public services were established. These new regimes included the creation of new regulatory bodies and inspection regimes for public bodies. For example, OFSTED became responsible for the inspection of schools, and subsequently children and families social work services. NPM requires what is termed a purchaser/provider split. In health and social care, this split was legally introduced by the NHS and Community Care Act (NHS and CC Act; House of Commons, 1990). The purchaser/provider split breaks up a monopoly of service provision. Social workers became care managers. The care manager role is a significantly different from the tradition social work role. A pure model of care management sees the care manager acting in a brokering role between service users and service providers. This was always an uneasy fit and the model did not transfer easily into the area of mental health social work. The NHS and CC Act (1990) and related policies were written in the language of consumer choice. One of the outcomes of NPM was the development of an audit culture. This involved the creation of bureaucracies to manage the data required to demonstrate how an organisation was performing against a series of Key Performance Indicators (KPIs). These changes have had a profound impact on the nature of the public sector. The inquiries that are discussed in this chapter have to be placed in the broader context of this development of a new form of organisational governmentality.

High profile cases such as the murder of Jonathan Zito by Christopher Clunis were reported in such as a way that they became to be seen as representative of the whole policy (Cummins, 2010b). The inquiry culture was part of the developing and ultimate dominant risk paradigm. The response to the failings of community care was a series of policies that were based on the auditing of professionals – marginalising relational approaches to work in mental health services. The media reporting of these inquiries had a particularly powerful impact in constructing a narrative that 'community care has failed'. This phrase was used by the then Secretary of State for Health, Frank Dobson, when he introduced New Labour's *Modernising Mental Health Services: Safe, Sound and Supportive* (Department of Health,

1999) – note the use of language here: supportive mental health services coming after safety.

Inquiry culture

Butler and Drakeford (2005) highlight the role that scandals have had in the broader development of British public policy. This seems to be particularly the case in the area of social work. Changes in social work practice and legislation have often been a response to high profile cases. In the area of children and families social work, a public inquiry in response to a high profile child death has been a recurring feature of the policy landscape for the past 70 years (Warner, 2015). In the area of mental health, a series of inquiries into institutional abuse played a key role in highlighting the abusive nature of the asylum regime. This is not just a recent phenomenon. One of the most famous psychiatric institutions in the UK – the York Retreat, established in 1796 – was a response to a scandal. In 1790, Hannah Mills, a local Quaker, died as the result of appalling neglect in the local lunatic asylum. William Tuke and other members of the Quaker community raised funds to establish the Retreat (Cummins, 2017). More recently the Ely Inquiry (Howe, 1969) into the abuse of patients at a large psychiatric unit outside Cardiff was prompted by allegations from a whistle blower. The allegations were originally made in a letter to the *News of the World*. The Inquiry was chaired by Geoffrey Howe, later Chancellor of the Exchequer, during the Thatcher administrations. The Ely report presented a picture of wider neglect – an institution that was representative of the wider isolation, geographical, psychological and professional of mental health services of the period. One part-time and two full-time doctors were responsible for the care of more than 660 patients. There were difficulties in recruiting staff to an institution whose buildings were over 100 years old.

There is something of a shift in focus in the mental health inquiries from the late 1980s onwards. There were inquiries that focused on institutional issues – for example, the Ashworth Inquiry headed by Louis Blom-Cooper (Department of Health, 1992) and the Fallon Inquiry (Fallon et al, 1999) into Lawrence Ward, the personality disorder unit at Ashworth. However, the majority of these inquiries and certainly the most high profile – the Ritchie Inquiry into the care and treatment of Christopher Clunis (Ritchie et al, 1994) – focused on cases of homicide committed by individuals either with a history of mental illness or recent contact with mental health services. The

'Spokes Inquiry' (DHSS, 1988) was established following the murder of Isabel Schwarz (1955–84), a psychiatric social worker based at Bexley Hospital. Schwarz was stabbed to death by Sharon Campbell, who was 20 years old. Campbell had previously been a patient at Bexley and had been discharged against her will. She had previously attacked Schwarz and made other threats against her. Schwarz was attacked when she was working at the hospital late one evening. The Inquiry highlighted a number of issues that became recurring themes of later cases – poor communication, lack of coordination between services and the failure to take a holistic view of the assessment of risk. Butler and Drakeford (2005) suggest that Schwarz's position as a social worker and the contradictory status that it has meant that this awful case did not become a scandal. The Inquiry recommended there should be a register of the most vulnerable mentally ill patients living in the community and they should be appointed keyworkers to have a coordinating role in their care (DHSS, 1988). The Spokes Inquiry led to the Griffiths Report (1988), the forerunner of the NHS and Community Care Act (1990).

Moral panics

Social work and social workers are often caught up in the moral panics of the day (Butler and Drakeford, 2005). On one level, this given the nature of social work and its liminal position between individuals, families, communities and the wider state, this is not surprising. There was a moral panic about the perceived failings of community care in the late 1980s and 1990s. Community care, in this context, was specifically used as a shorthand for mental health services – other areas of provision were not subject to such scrutiny or detailed media coverage. Cohen's (1972) notion of a moral panic provides a theoretical lens through which the responses to inquiries into homicides, committed by those with current or some previous contact with mental health services, can be explored. *Policing the Crisis* (Hall et al, 2013) is a classic study of the way that moral panics reflect wider social and political disquiet. Its discussion of the way that racialised narratives have a key role in many moral panics is important in the mental health field. Hall et al (2013) seek to explore how and why particular themes, including crime and other deviant acts, produce such a reaction. They argue that social and moral issues are much more likely to be the source of these panics. There are certain areas, for example youth culture, drugs or lone parents, where there are recurring panics. The response to this panic includes not only societal control mechanisms, such as the courts, but also the media becoming an important mediating agency between the state and the formation of public opinion.

There have been a series of moral panics following the deaths of children. Jones (2014) shows the role that the media played in demonising social workers in the aftermath of the death of 'Baby P'. Warner (2015) highlights that politicians had a key, often inflammatory, role in the developing media coverage. David Cameron and Ed Balls both wrote emotive newspaper columns about the case. In these columns, both politicians made links between their own experiences as fathers and their disgust at the treatment inflicted on 'Baby P'. Of course, one does not have to be a parent to be repulsed by neglect and abuse of a child. Cameron and Balls were doing this to side with 'ordinary' members of the public as opposed to 'out of touch' social workers who, in this narrative, had allowed these events to occur.

In *Policing the Crisis* (Hall et al, 2013) explores the development of a moral panic that focused on street robberies – muggings – in the mid-1970s. The media reporting of these crimes is examined. Hall et al (2013) interest was initially triggered by the sentencing of a local youth to 20 years for such an offence. The reports of these crimes were racialised in the sense that the media presented mugging as a 'black crime'. Hall was working in Birmingham and the impact of Enoch Powell's 'Rivers of Blood' speech cast a long shadow (Hirsch, 2018). Powell in his speech had claimed that one of his elderly constituents was trapped in her home because of the fear of being attacked by local black youths.

In his consideration of Hall, Simon (2014) notes that muggings were not the most pressing social or crime problem that communities faced in this period. This was a period that saw the advanced industrial economies entering a decade long period of almost continuous recession and inflation. Alongside this, a period of deindustrialisation was underway which would see the UK economy become dominated by the financial services sector. This included a further shift of economic and political power to London and the south of the country (Simon, 2014). In addition, the early 1970s was a period of huge political turmoil in the UK. This included industrial conflict – there were miners strikes in 1972 and 1974. The Heath government introduced a three-day week to protect energy supplies between December 1973 and February 1974 (Wheen, 2009). 1972 was the bloodiest year of the Troubles in Northern Ireland (McKittrick and McVea, 2001) when 479 people were killed and 4,876 injured.

The factors outlined here lead Hall et al (2013) to argue that the state faced a crisis of legitimacy. 'Black crime' became a signifier used by the media and politicians to represent the social problems in what Hall and his colleagues termed 'urban colonies'. They used this term as a radical alternative to other phrases used at the time such as ghetto or inner-city. These terms were, also, racially coded. The folk devil of the urban crime moral panic of the early 1970s was a black youth. Moral panics lead to calls for action. Violent crime tends to generate powerful support for state responses – more police officers, longer custodial sentences and harsher conditions in prisons. Hall et al (2013) show the way that the strong state uses 'law and order' policies to generate support from working class and middle class voters.

This study is remarkably prescient in that it describes the way that the politics of law and order developed in the years following its publication. The Criminal Justice System (CJS) has historically been one of the key sites of social work interventions (Cummins, 2017). The rise of managerialism has marginalised social work approaches in the CJS. The focus is on risk and risk management (Garland, 2001, 2004). The 'othering' of other social groups – poor, marginalised, urban communities and minorities – is both a cause and an outcome of increased inequality. It is one of the key drivers of increased punitivism (Garland, 2001, 2004). Hall et al (2013) demonstrate that an expansion of the penal state is a key feature of the New Right thinking, which is a combination of economic liberalism and social conservatism. Modern discourses of penal policy create an often racialised image of the offender as an alien – someone who is 'not one of us'. This approach also provides valuable insights into the way that particular cases were given a high profile in the reporting of community care (Cummins, 2010b).

Christopher Clunis

The importance of representation has been discussed in the previous section. The photograph of Christopher Clunis that has been reproduced so many times since 1994 plays on several racial stereotypes but also those of mental illness. Cross (2010) notes that there is a long standing trope that focuses on the physicality of the mentally ill. This is partly a Gothic notion whereby wild hair, exaggerated strength and other physical signs represent not only the inner turmoil of madness but also the threat that is allegedly posed to the wider society. There is an overlap here between this and the long standing racist stereotype of the large physically aggressive black man. In this context, it is important to provide some background details that a picture of Clunis's life before that photograph was taken.

Christopher Clunis was born in Muswell Hill, London in 1963. He did well at school and obtained six O levels. He began A levels, but he left to pursue a career in music. He found work on in bands on cruise ships. After the publication of the Ritchie inquiry, the owner of a music shop wrote to the Audit Commission Inquiry into community care, with his memories of Clunis. These were of a talented musician, who was a regular customer at his shop, a quiet rather unassuming character. He had no recollection of Clunis being violent and was shocked by the newspaper reports of the murder of Jonathan Zito. While he was working on a cruise ship, Clunis's parents returned to Jamaica as his mother suffered a stroke. She died in 1985 when Clunis was on tour. It was some time before the family could contact him with the news and he missed the funeral. From 1986 onwards, Clunis's mental state seems to have deteriorated significantly. His personal care was poor, and he began to dress in a bizarre fashion. He went to stay with a sister, but he had to leave when he hit his niece. As the family struggled to support him, he moved to live with his father in Jamaica. It was during this period that he was first admitted to a psychiatric unit – Bellevue Hospital in Kingston.

In 1987, Clunis returned to live in London. It is this period up until his arrest for the murder of Jonathan Zito, a complete stranger to him, that is detailed in the report. The murder took place at Finsbury Park tube station in December 1992. It is the period between 1987 and 1992 that is covered in the Inquiry. Clunis's mental health deteriorated to the extent that he was admitted to hospital in June 1987. The Inquiry then outlines a pattern of relatively short admissions to hospital. He was admitted four times under the Mental Health Act (MHA) prior to December 1992. These admissions to hospital followed by an early discharge without adequate support followed by periods of homelessness or living in bed and breakfasts (B&Bs) and hostels. The Inquiry states that Clunis had a history of sexually disinhibited and violent behaviour. There were several assaults on staff and other patients – including threats with knives and a screwdriver. At no point in this five-year period were agencies able to engage successfully with Clunis. In December 1993, he was convicted of manslaughter on the grounds of diminished responsibility.

The Inquiry

The establishment of the Inquiry was due to the campaigning of Jayne Zito, Jonathan's widow. The *Independent* newspaper had also carried out an investigation into the case, publishing an article about it in July 1993.

The terms of reference of the Inquiry were:

1. to investigate all the circumstances surrounding the admission, treatment, discharge and continuing care of Christopher Clunis between May 1992 and December 1992;
2. to identify any deficiencies in the quality and delivery of that care, as well as interagency collaboration and individual responsibilities; and
3. to make recommendations for the future delivery of care including admission, treatment, discharge and continuing care to people in similar circumstances so that, as far as possible, harm to patients and the public is avoided.

After some initial work, the Inquiry decided to extend its remit so that it examined a longer period than the six months prior to the murder of Jonathan Zito. This has the advantage of providing a more detailed complex picture of Clunis's contact with mental health services. However, one of the dangers of the Inquiry culture, as previously discussed, is the inherent hindsight bias. The danger is that the events that led up to the homicide or tragic event are seen as inevitable. Thus all other contacts are then read through a prism that we know that an individual has committed a very serious crime. Warner (2006) highlights the importance and attraction of this narrative structure. It generates the notion – more prevalent in child death inquiries – that there were missed opportunities where agencies could and should have acted differently. The logic being that this would have prevented a particular outcome. This is not to defend poor practice or to argue that we should not examine such cases. It is rather to suggest that such an approach inevitably leads to the scapegoating of individuals and a failure to look at systemic and organisational issues. The Ritchie Inquiry includes examples of poor practice – for example inadequate discharge planning. In one case, a professional was appointed Section 117 key worker for Clunis. The Section 117 discharge meeting had taken place across the other side of London and the key worker was not present at the meeting. This is clearly indefensible, but the decision should be placed in an organisational context. The Inquiry report also includes examples of practitioners working against the odds in underfunded and overstretched services.

Apart from two short periods in 1988 and 1989, the final report provides a detailed history of Clunis's contact with the mental health and CJS systems. In the period between June 1987 and December 1992, he was admitted to hospital on ten occasions. He was assessed by 30 psychiatrists. The report details his contact with the CJS, which included three remands into custody. Clunis lived in five different hostels and six B&Bs. These stays were usually ended because of violent or socially unacceptable behaviour on Clunis's part. Coid (1994) notes that Clunis moved across London, whether by accident or design is not clear. It meant that he was moving from one team to another and there was no continuity of care. At the time of the homicide of Jonathan Zito, Clunis was living alone in a bedsit, which was dirty and cold. The police when they searched it found unused medication and appointment letters from mental health and social work staff.

Coid (1994), an experienced consultant psychiatrist, concluded that the Ritchie Inquiry was right in many of its observations and conclusions, particularly about the lack of secure forensic mental health provision in London at that time. He is also critical of the way that the issue of Clunis's violent history was downplayed. Coid (1994) felt that the Inquiry highlighted the way that mental health services were reluctant to engage in a more assertive fashion with patients who presented in this fashion. He notes that this is a small group but argued that there was a need for a shift in approach, including the introduction of community treatment orders in some form, as well as attitudes within services. He concluded that

> The legislation which might have ensured some chance of his receiving treatment outside of hospital does not exist. Furthermore, the type of in-patient facility that he truly needed has been closed in much of the UK. If ever a patient required prolonged institutional care it was Clunis. Sadly, it was only after he killed an innocent member of the public that he could receive it. (Coid, 1994: 452)

The issue of race and psychiatry remains a controversial one. Coid (1994) notes that the Ritchie Inquiry notes that there was a tendency to overlook or minimise Christopher Clunis's significant history of violent behaviour. In addition, the report concluded those responsible for his care avoided difficult decisions because Clunis was 'and possibly because he was big and black'. Cummins (2015) explores the way that issues of race are addressed in the Ritchie Inquiry (Ritchie et al, 1994) and the Prins Inquiry report (1993) entitled *Big, Black and Dangerous*, which was published in the same period. The Prins Inquiry was established following the death of Orville Blackwood at Broadmoor Special Hospital. Blackwood's death was the third of an African-Caribbean male patient. He died after being restrained and heavily medicated. The Prins Inquiry is forthright in its criticisms of the way that the Broadmoor regime of the time failed to engage with issues of race. The report concluded that 'the interpretation is based on some very crude measures of racism' – for example, reported incidents of direct racial abuse or the use of racial epithets. Many of the features of a modern public service, such as an Equal Opportunities policy, ethnic monitoring and service user involvement, were missing. The hospital did not even collect basic information such as the number of black patients. The phrase 'big, black and dangerous' is a shorthand that the Inquiry uses for the ways in which Orville Blackwood and other black patients were viewed. It is not a phrase that the Inquiry invented; it was one that was openly used among nursing staff.

The Ritchie Inquiry (Ritchie et al, 1994) is much more circumspect. The Inquiry team were unable to find any evidence that racial prejudice or discrimination had any impact on the care and treatment Clunis received – apart from some staff were too willing to accept that he abused drugs. At this distance, this appears a very partial analysis or view of what might be considered prejudice or discrimination. The example given by the report is, of course, one of the most persistent stereotypes of young black men. Cannabis induced psychosis was one of the main hypothesis that sought to explain the overrepresentation of African-Caribbean men in mental health services in this period (Sharpley et al, 2001) The issue here does not relate to whether an individual patient did or did not use drugs. It is rather whether mental health professionals formed a particular view based on stereotypical views and without evidence.

One of the most shocking areas of both reports is the treatment of the relatives of the two men. This reflects a series of long held historical views that pathologises the 'black family'. In the case of Christopher Clunis, as the Ritchie Inquiry (1994, para 3.1.6.) puts it: 'They treated him as single, homeless and itinerant with no family ties, the more they treated him as such the more he began to fulfil that role.' There were few attempts, even though he had been detained under the MHA, to contact Clunis's sister. The fact he had a sister and she had been in regular contact with him was ignored. The Prins Inquiry was shocked by the treatment of the Blackwood family. There were no clear procedures for informing the family. When his mother eventually was able to see her son's body, it was in a refrigerator at the mortuary. She was able to see other bodies at the same time. The Inquiry panel visited the mortuary to confirm that this was the case.

The marginalisation of family members and the refusal to be open about the events that led to their loved one's death has been a feature of the authorities' responses in such cases. Joan Bennett, the sister of Rocky Bennett, campaigned vigorously for a public inquiry into her brother's death. Rocky died in circumstances not unlike those of Orville Blackwood being restrained by staff while a patient in a secure psychiatric facility (Blofeld, 2004). The Ritchie Inquiry (1994) does not engage with the idea that racism by individuals or organisations may have had an impact on the care or treatment that Christopher Clunis received. It seems unsustainable to believe that race played no part at all in the failure of services or that Clunis never encountered racist behaviour (Cummins, 2015).

Inquiries in context

Public inquiries have been something of a standard response to major controversies across a range of events. In recent years, we have seen the Hutton Inquiry into the Iraq War, the Saville Inquiry into Bloody Sunday and the Francis Inquiry into Mid-Staffs hospital. There have been a number of high profile social work related inquiries over the past 30 years. In the mid-1990s, there were increasing concerns about the failings in community care including a rise in the number of homeless people but also a series of homicides involving people who had some form of contact with mental health services. The government circulars HSG (94)27 and LASSL (94)4 'Guidance on the discharge of mentally disordered people and their continuing care in the community' made such inquiries a statutory requirement in cases of homicide where there was contact with mental health services (Department of Health, 1994). The circular also established supervision registers which are discussed in the next paragraph.

HSG (94)27 emphasised the need for thorough and ongoing assessment of those patients considered to present the most significant risks. In a section headed 'If things go wrong' it is made clear that in cases of homicide there should be, after the completion of legal proceedings, an independent inquiry. The remit of the inquiry is to examine at least the following:

- the care the patient was receiving at the time of the incident;
- the suitability of that care in view of the patient's assessed health and social care needs;
- the extent to which that care corresponded with statutory obligations, relevant guidance from the Department of Health and local operational policies;
- the exercise of professional judgement;
- the adequacy of the care plan and its monitoring by the key worker.

The guidance also addressed the composition of the inquiry panel and the distribution of reports. It stated 'consideration should be given to appointing a lawyer as chairman' – this became standard practice. Two of the most high profile inquiries, for example, into the Clunis case and the care and treatment of Andrew Robinson were headed by QCs – Jean Ritchie and Louis Blom-Cooper. Other members of the panel were to include a psychiatrist and a senior social services manager or senior nurse. A formal requirement to publish the final report was not established. However, there was a requirement to make the main findings 'available to interested parties'. Prins (2004), in discussing inquiries generally, noted that only a limited number of copies of the final inquiry report *Big, Black and Dangerous* were printed.

The late Louis Blom-Cooper conducted not only community inquiries but also chaired an inquiry at Ashworth Hospital. He had been chair of the panel that produced *A Child in Trust, the Report of the Panel of Inquiry into the Circumstances surrounding the Death of Jasmine Beckford* (Blom-Cooper, 1985). Blom-Cooper (1999) argued that the purpose of any inquiry was to establish the truth – what happened, how did it happen and whether any professional was culpable. He also suggested the inquiry process can provide some form of public catharsis. The inquiry can look at material that would not come before a court in the legal proceedings so can provide some answers to families and carers. In addition, there is the hope that such inquiries will be able to provide wider lessons for mental health professionals. Inquiries quickly became embedded within the mental health landscape. The Royal College of Psychiatrists (RCP, 1996) noted that there were 39 homicides covering at two periods totalling 26 months. All related to offences committed by patients who had had contact with mental health services in the 12 months. There were only nine inquiries between 1988 and 1994 (Sheppard, 1995). There were 27 published in 1997 and 1998 (Sheppard, 1998).

RCP (1996) produced a summary of the key themes that emerged from a series of inquiries. These can be summarised as:

- key problem areas;
- failures in communication;
- poor and unclear care plans;
- lack of direct contact with patients;
- gaps in staff training;
- poor compliance with medication;
- understanding and use of legal powers under the MHA.

The RCP report's recommendations included:

- improved risk assessment;
- more direct contact with patients;
- improving wards;
- MHA training for staff;
- better communication systems – between professionals but also between professionals and families;
- the development of genuine multi-disciplinary teams.

In later inquiries, there were recommendations for reform of the MHA including the introduction of a form of community treatment order.

Coppock and Hopton (2002) note that the inquiry culture, by focusing on specific cases, inevitably produces a narrative of local individual rather than systemic failures. The more fundamental issues and fissures in community care that exist at a policy level – the lack of adequate funding, the complex organisational structure, the impact of professional hierarchies and a legal framework that was based on the asylum system – become marginalised or even totally ignored. Stanley and Manthorpe (2001) argue that inquiries focus on the failure of services to police risky individuals rather than organisational and structural issues. The only inquiry that did this in the period was the Audit Commission's (1994) *Finding A Place*. This document starts from a values-based approach rather than an organisational one – it asks the fundamental question what the core of mental health services should be. It has a focus on service user views and needs that is largely missing from the other inquiries discussed here. These core values such as respect and support then form the building blocks for the structure of services.

Inquiries were criticised for being too costly and time consuming. In addition, the process was part of the creation of a blame culture. Organisations and industries, for example the airline industry, which have created a more open culture to address safety issues have recognised the importance of examining all cases where things go wrong. This includes 'near misses'. It also requires that all staff at any level are encouraged to raise potential issues. Reith (1998) in an analysis of inquiry reports emphasised that this was not a luxury but a necessity. It is, of course, somewhat easier said than done. The hierarchical nature of the medical profession is clearly a factor. Stanley and Manthorpe (2001) highlight the dangers of hindsight bias in the inquiry process. Inquiries placed huge emphasise on the importance of chronologies – a key feature of risk assessment being a detailed history. This is not that surprising as it is the role of the inquiry. However, there is an inherent danger in working backwards from the homicide that triggered the inquiry. If the homicide had not occurred, then there would not have been an inquiry. This does not mean that the structural and other issues highlighted in the final report did not exist.

Warner (2006) argues that inquiries are 'active texts' (Prior, 2003). They have to be examined in the social and political context in which they were created and written. She highlights that the inquiries in this period had a vital role in the construction of a narrative that linked the asylum closure programme – which had been underway for 30 years at this point – to alleged increases in violent offences committed by mentally ill perpetrators. One of the most important aspects of the influence of inquiries is the way that they were reported in the media. The general public and, in truth, most professionals will only see media reports of most inquiries. Even the reports of the most high profile ones are not widely read in full. This is partly an issue of time and work pressures. There is also a form of groupthink that all inquiries say the same things – this is far from the case. Newspaper and TV coverage is inevitably a partial rendering of the complexity of the issues discussed in the final report. Warner (2006) stated there was an intertextual relationship between the reports and media accounts that was a key factor in the creation of a blame culture.

Psychiatrists were particularly critical of these processes. Muijen (1996) saw inquiries failing either to reassure the public or improve mental health systems. The consultant psychiatrist George Szmulker (2000) wrote a reflective piece about his involvement in the Inquiry into the care of Luke Warm Luke (Scotland, 1998). Michael Folkes, 32, who had changed his name to Luke Warm Luke, murdered his partner Susan Crawford. To emphasise Warner's (2006) point about the intertextuality of media and inquiry reports – the *Independent* (1998) article on the publication of the report was headlined 'Schizophrenic visited clinic before killing'. It went on to say:

> Despite a history of violence, he had been allowed to live alone and take responsibility for his own medication. The killing happened eight hours after a doctor had put Luke on a list for emergency attention. He turned up in a distressed state at the Maudsley hospital on 3 October 1994, but was allowed to leave.

Szmulker is clearly not an impartial observer. He is open about this. He points out that the Inquiry took four years and cost in the region of £750,000. Szmulker (2000) argues that the inquiry culture rather than reassuring the public has increased fears that they will be killed by a psychotic stranger. The risks of this are 1 in 10 million. This case was like others in that those at greatest risk are family and carers. Szmulker (2000) concludes that the inquiries reinforced a spurious relationship between community care and homicides. A form of community care hindsight bias (Hawkins and Hastie, 1990) developed, which assumed that these cases could be prevented by good services or by professionals following the procedures and policies as they currently existed. This is far too strong a claim (Szmulker, 2000). The process is also a traumatic one for the family and friends of both the victim and the perpetrator – often these groups can overlap. The publication is potentially the third or fourth time that the case has received media coverage – the initial homicide, reports that the perpetrator is mentally ill, the court case and finally a press conference. The final area to consider is the impact on staff morale both in the long and the short term.

Prins (1998) argued that the development of the mental health inquiry system should be placed in the wider context of the CJS. The inquiries were related to offending rather than solely mental health issues. Prins (1998) is referring to the development of a newly punitive approach. Faulkner (1997) saw society becoming more exclusionary. One of the major concerns of mental health professionals was that they were being asked to take on a role that was more appropriate for their criminal justice colleagues. This mistakenly assumes that there are concrete barriers between the two systems (Seddon, 2009). One of the most important issues in these debates is the nature of the links between mental illness and offending – particularly homicide.

National Confidential Inquiry

In 1992, the National Confidential Inquiry into Suicides and Homicides by People with Mental Illness (NCI) was established. It has been based at the University of Manchester since 1996. The Inquiry was established with two major aims:

- To establish the frequency and contributory role of mental illness in a complete national sample of homicides.
- To examine aggregate data on those in contact with mental health services to inform clinical practice and policy.

This thematic approach would answer key questions about the rate of homicide among those with mental illness but also provide an analysis of risk factors. The NCI is thus a step removed from the initial inquiries that were the source of such personal and professional angst for many involved in mental health services. Shaw et al (2006) carried out a clinical survey of people who were convicted of homicide in England and Wales in the period 1996–99. This is the period when there were several inquiries. This study examined 1,594 convictions for homicide in that period: 545 (34 per cent) of perpetrators experienced some form of mental disorder but the majority had not been in contact with psychiatric services; 85 (5 per cent) had a schizophrenia; and 164 (10 per cent) experienced symptoms at the time of the offence. In these cases, verdict of diminished responsibility was returned in 149 (9 per cent). The Court imposed a hospital order in 111 (7 per cent) of cases. The most common method of killing was stabbing and this occurred in 594 (37 per cent) of cases. The survey reported that the relationship between the perpetrator and the victim was recorded in 1,432 of these homicides: 511 (36 per cent) involved the homicide of a family member including current or former spouses or partners; 563 (39 per cent) cases involved the homicide of a friend or acquaintance; 358 (25 per cent) were cases of stranger attacks. Shaw et al (2006: 146) concluded that:

> ... most perpetrators with a history of mental disorder were not acutely ill when they killed and most had never received mental healthcare, suggesting that services could not have prevented their offences.

Swinson et al (2011) reported findings from an analysis of 5,884 homicides notified to the NCI for the period 1997–2006. In this cohort, there were 605 (10 per cent) cases where the perpetrator exhibited some symptoms of mental disorder at the time of the offence; and 598 (10 per cent) had had some recent contact with mental health services. In 331 (6 per cent) cases, there was evidence that the perpetrator exhibited psychotic symptoms at the time of the offence. The authors suggest that the increase in the prevalence of psychosis may be down to more prevalent drug misuse which might have triggered symptoms. The NCI has played a key role in highlighting the need to be very cautious when making claims about links between mental illness and violent crime generally and homicides. We need to take a much broader view. The overwhelming majority of homicides are impulsive and unplanned acts. Crichton (2011) carried out a review of 236 inquiries published between 1995 and 2010. These involved the homicides of 252 victims. He concluded that the inquiries typically about cases where a man, usually in his twenties or thirties, stabbed a family member with a kitchen knife. The victim was often a carer or family member who lived with the perpetrator. One harm reduction method would be taking action to limit access to kitchen knives. This is not to diminish the significance of these cases or the traumatic impact on families. It is rather to ask questions about what services might have done differently.

Mental health inquiries do not occupy the prominent media position that they once did. The moral panic of the 1990s had passed and other issues in the area of mental health policy have a prominent profile. The more recent focus has been on the reform of the MHA and wider pressures on services (Cummins, 2019). However, it would be a mistake to think that a) homicides involving individuals with a history of mental illness or contact with services do not take place; or b) there is not an official investigation. Such events are much more likely to gain local rather than national coverage. From April 2013 NHS England became responsible for commissioning independent investigations into such homicides. These inquiries are now carried out by independent consultancy agencies – the consultants are usually former senior nursing or social care professionals. The remit of these investigations is slightly different to the inquiries examined here. However, the purpose of the investigation is to review thoroughly the care and treatment of the patient.

The aim is that the NHS can:

- be clear about what – if anything – went wrong with the care of the patient;
- minimise the possibility of a reoccurrence of similar events;
- make recommendations for the delivery of health services in the future.

The investigation team has access to all the information and reports about the individual patient's care and treatment, and can also request interviews with any NHS staff involved. In the North of England region, there were 46 such investigations in between 2013 and 2018.

Conclusion

This chapter has examined the key role that inquiries played in community care in the late 1980s and early 1990s. In this area, the Ritchie Inquiry (1994) is a key document because of the extensive media coverage that it received. Warner (2006) terms it an 'index' inquiry because of its significance. Inquiries had a key role in the construction of a particular narrative of community care – that became the dominant one – the narrative was that the system had failed. It should be emphasised that these were not presented as individual catastrophic failures. They were presented as systemic failures – though ironically few inquiries gave any real consideration to the broader issues in the development of community care. The only area to receive a detailed focus in recommendations was the issue of reform of the MHA. The eventual introduction of Community Treatment Orders (CTOs) was, in no small part, due to the recommendations in these inquiries that there needed to be some way of ensuring that patients who had been discharged from hospital took medication. Other issues such as housing, employment, racism and stigma were much more marginal. The voices of service users, families and carers are largely absent from the inquiry discourse.

The policy responses such as supervision registers were based on a fundamental belief that the solutions to the issues raised by inquiries the problems were to be found in a legislative framework rather than the organisation, structure and delivery of services. CTOs developed something of a mythic status during this period becoming seen as a solution to all the issues raised. However, we should note here that, in the overwhelming majority of cases that led to an Inquiry, the patient had the right to Section 117 MHA aftercare because they had been detained under Section 3 MHA 1983. There was a duty on health and social services to provide this aftercare. This is not to minimise the potential difficulties of working in overstretched services. It is simply to question whether the legislation was the key factor. If we take the case of Christopher Clunis, if CTOs had existed in 1989–90 he would have almost certainly been subject to one. One is forced to ask did (or do) the services exist to effectively enact such legislation. For example, it would have been difficult to recall him if there was not a hospital bed.

Inquiries and the tabloid media reporting helped to support a view that one of the causes of the failings of mental health policy was the increased rights being afforded to patients (Cummins, 2010b). This was before the introduction of the Human Rights Act and in a period of Conservative governments which, up to 1992, had significant Commons majorities. The notion here is that agencies were refusing to act, particularly on the concerns expressed by families, because of mental health professionals' liberal commitment to patients' rights. I am aware that many service users might struggle with the platonic idealism of a liberal mental health professional with a commitment to patients' rights. Psychiatry seemed to have moved from being criticised as an agent of social control to neglecting this aspect of its function.

Szmulker (2000) noted that the plethora of media reports about these inquiries added to the general public disquiet about community care. The media reported, often in lurid terms, these events on such a regular basis that public perceptions of the risk were increased. These were out of all proportion to the actual risks. Beck (1992) highlights that this is one of the features of the risk society. The government was never able or willing to mount a sustained defence of the policy of community care. Far from creating an open culture where professionals, alongside service users, families and carers, are able to discuss risks and how services should respond, inquiries did the opposite. Mental health services and professionals felt that they were being asked to take responsibility for the issue of violent crime. The result was that managerialism rather than the progressive values of community care began to dominate.

5

Deinstitutionalisation and the penal state

Introduction

The increase in the use of imprisonment is referred to by penal scholars by a variety of terms, such as 'mass incarceration' or 'the penal state'. These terms capture the shift that has occurred since the early 1980s whereby rates of imprisonment have almost doubled in some countries. The US led the way in the expansion of the use of imprisonment. There are now more than 2 million Americans in custody. The overwhelming majority of prisoners – as in all countries – come from poor, urban communities. Racial minorities are overrepresented (Simon, 2007; Clear, 2009; Alexander, 2012). These developments in the penal system have taken place during a period when mental health institutions have closed. This chapter will explore the relationship between deinstitutionalisation and the increase in the use of imprisonment. The chapter begins with a consideration of the problem of how we define 'mentally disordered offenders'. There is then a brief outline of the Penrose Hypothesis (Penrose, 1939; 1943), which sought to explain the links between the use of imprisonment and institutionalised psychiatric care. This approach will be used as a critical lens through which to examine policy developments in this area. Broader issues regarding the treatment of mentally disordered offenders will then be discussed. This section will highlight the pressures on the Criminal Justice System (CJS) and the way that it has become, in many cases, a de facto provider of mental health care. The argument that deinstitutionalisation has led to the 'criminalisation of the mentally ill' will be discussed. The legacy of deinstitutionalisation and the expansion of the penal state will be discussed, focusing on contemporary issues in the CJS.

The problem of definition

What do we mean by the term 'mentally disordered offender'? At first, this appears a straightforward question: surely it is an offender who has committed offences as a result of the symptoms of mental illness. However, further consideration reveals that the complexities of the debates in this field. A very narrow definition of the term might limit its use to those who had been convicted and sentenced under the provisions of the Mental Health Act (1983). This is actually a very small group indeed. Such a definition would exclude important areas where the CJS and mental health systems intersect. For example, people with mental health problems who are in contact with the police either because of a mental health crisis or because they are in custody would not be included.

The use of the term 'offender' is also problematic. An offender is someone who has been convicted of an offence. Someone is detained under Section 136 MHA by a police officer because of concerns about their welfare – not because of suspicions that they have committed an offence. However, they have been drawn into the CJS by virtue of their contact with the police. The limited research that explores the experiences of people detained under Section 136 indicates that it is regarded as a punitive rather than therapeutic intervention (Riley et al, 2011). It is important that in this area we do not use a definition that would, perhaps, unintentionally exclude significant numbers of people. A very broad definition is required. This might require ceasing to use terms such as 'mentally disordered offender' or limiting its use to very specific circumstances. A broader term such as 'people with mental health problems in contact with the CJS' attempts to capture the variety and complex of the groups involved. This definition acknowledges the porous nature of the boundaries between the CJS and mental health systems. Law and policy allow that the mental health of an individual can and should be a consideration in decisions at every stage of the CJS. This is the case from potential contact with a police officer on the street, through custody, charging and sentencing. The police, courts and prisons can be viewed as a series of filters (Cummins, 2016).

The Penrose Hypothesis

Lionel Penrose (1898–1972) was a British geneticist who undertook research into schizophrenia and Down's syndrome. Penrose was from a Quaker family, educated at Quaker schools and St John's College, Cambridge. He was a conscientious objector in the First World War and served with the Friends' Ambulance Unit in France. In his work on genetics, Penrose identified the chromosomal causes of learning disabilities. In addition, Penrose put forward a hypothesis that argued that there was a link between rates of imprisonment and the use of institutionalised forms of psychiatric care. In two papers (Penrose, 1939;

1943), he argued that there is an essentially fluid relationship between the two. The first paper is a statistical analysis of rates of imprisonment and psychiatric institutionalisation in European countries. It identified an inverse relationship between the provision of mental hospitals and the rate of serious crime in the countries studied – as one increases, the other decreases. The 1943 paper was a study of the rates of hospital admission in different states in the US and the numbers in state prisons. Penrose suggested that it would be possible to produce an 'index of development' for each country. This would be obtained by dividing the total number of people in mental hospitals and similar institutions by the number of people in prison.

The relationship between the policies of deinstitutionalisation and the development of the penal state will now be examined in more detail. On the surface, there appears to be a great deal of evidence to support the main thrust of Penrose's arguments. The rates of imprisonment in countries such as England and Wales increased dramatically during periods when the number of mental health beds fell significantly. Research has highlighted the fact that offenders as a group have much higher rates of mental illness than other populations (Singleton et al 1998, Birmingham, 2003; 2004, Steel et al, 2007). This appears to hold across all groups of offenders. The CJS has become in many cases a de facto provider of mental health care (Cummins, 2016). However, the relationships between these two trends are complex.

At the core of the Penrose Hypothesis is an idea that society responds to certain forms of deviance by medicalising it or punishing it. In some cases, it does both. One critical reading of Penrose would be that he makes the mistake of equating mental illness with criminality. In opposing this view, I would argue that Penrose was making a case for more therapeutic interventions. His proposed index of development is a measure of the use of such approaches. It should be noted that Penrose's index is based on positive assumptions about the nature of an institutional regime to be therapeutic that many such as Goffman (2014) would come to dispute. The development of community based mental health services is based on both moral and clinical arguments. Its main proponents, for example, Basaglia in Italy, saw the institutionalised treatment of the mentally ill as a political issue, one of human rights (Foot, 2015; Cummins, 2018). Community based services, it was argued, would be more humane. These arguments are based on notions of citizenship. They assumed that community care services would be value driven. Those who argued for community based mental health services did not envisage that asylums would be replaced by police and prison cells. While he was not necessarily an advocate of community care, Penrose's work provided an important perspective. This perspective can be used to explore the development of CJS and mental health policies and the way that they intersect. In using the Penrose Hypothesis in this way, the work can be used a moral argument rather than a statistical analysis.

The CJS and mental health systems are often presented as two rather distinct systems that overlap in certain specific areas, such as forensic mental health services or the Police and Criminal Evidence Act (2004), which provides additional protections to people with mental health problems if they are in police custody. This two-systems approach is one that Penrose adopted when he developed this hypothesis. The reality on the ground is much messier and complex. Prisons and psychiatric institutions have always been used as a means to exclude and discipline individuals who are regarded as deviant in some way by the wider society (Foucault, 2003). The definitions of deviant, criminal and so on change over time, reflecting wider social, cultural and political values.

There is a danger of presentism in all areas of social policy. There are two elements to this. One is to ignore the historical roots of a policy. Questions about how we ended up in a situation are not simply of academic interest. They can often provide some guidance as to how to navigate a way out of the impasse. Another danger is that we see all problems as somehow new, unique to our current society or ones that have never been considered in the past. Finally, there is a danger that we ignore the errors of the past. Presentism is a potential trap, particularly in the criminal justice and mental health fields. John Howard carried out his famous inspection of the prisons in the 1780s. Modern readers may well be shocked by his description of the physical conditions, disease and hunger and the corruption among warders and how much of this is familiar. Howard (1780) also observed that there were more what he termed 'idiots and lunatics' in the prisons of the time. Howard highlighted that this increase meant that prison regimes were struggling to cope. Similar observations have been made ever since. The recent expansion in the use of imprisonment has occurred during the period when the impact of deinstitutionalisation has been most clearly felt.

The rise of the penal state

This section will provide a brief overview of the expansion the use of imprisonment. As noted, there are a number of terms that appear in the literature that used to describe this phenomenon: mass incarceration, mass imprisonment, the prison boom, the carceral state or the penal state. In summary, they all are used to describe the developments in social policy that have seen the increased use of prison, probation and community sanctions. These developments have occurred in a period when very broadly crime rates have been falling. The US has led the way in this penal arms race. Therefore, much of the analysis of this punitive turn has explored US policy. The expansion of the use of imprisonment has been a feature of several jurisdictions. Having outlined the rise of the penal state, I will then go to explore the intersection between penal and mental health policy. This analysis will use Penrose's Hypothesis as a conceptual framework for an exploration of these trends.

Simon (2014) in his discussion of the case of *Brown v. Plata,* compared the expansion of the use of imprisonment to a biblical flood. In *Brown v. Plata*, prisoners in California won a class action the state, suing on the basis of the conditions in prison. The overcrowding and inadequate healthcare for both physical and mental health issues was a breach of the 8th amendment. This is the constitutional prohibition on the use of cruel and unusual punishment. Simon (2007) sees the rise of the penal state in three interrelated phases. The fear of crime and the potential political fallout from being 'weak' on crime leads prosecutors to seek custodial sentences rather than community sentences. These custodial sentences are increased driven by continuing fears about the nature of violent crime and a belief that 'prison works'. Penal solutions for wider social problems become more popular or seen as the only option. The so-called *War on Drugs* is the perfect example of these processes. Finally, mandatory and or indeterminate sentences are introduced. Simon (2007), in discussing the political implications of these developments, noted that law and order has become a much more electorally significant issue. The centre ground of these debates has moved to the right, forcing progressive parties – in the words of Tony Blair – to become 'tough on crime, tough on the causes of crime'.

The standard comparative measure for imprisonment is the rate per 100,000 of the population. Since 1999, the overall world prison population rate has increased from 136 per 100,000 to 144 per 100,000. The US remains at the top of this incarceration league with a rate of 716 per 100,000. This average hides huge disparities between individual states. Carson and Golinelli's (2013) analysis showed that the five states with highest imprisonment rates – Louisiana (1,720), Mississippi (1,370) Alabama (1,234) Oklahoma (1,178) and Texas (1,121) – have rates well above the national average. If they were separate countries, they would have the highest rates of imprisonment in the world. Individuals are imprisoned but the impact is far wider than that. The rise of the penal state has inflicted huge collateral damage on the African-American community (Mauer, 2006; Clear, 2009; Drucker, 2011). The damage does not end when individuals are released. Many US states prevent ex-prisoners from voting, accessing social housing or completing educational programmes. Alexander (2012) powerfully argues that the overall effect creates a new 'caste' of disenfranchised and marginalised young black men. There is now a significant social grass roots movement that is challenging the expansion of the penal state — framing it as an issue of civil rights. The focus is not just on the use of imprisonment but also conditions within the systems. The Oscar nominated documentary film *13th* which highlighted these issues received wide coverage. The 13th amendment to the US Constitution abolished slavery but there was an exception for prisoners. The film highlights the racism of the current system.

In Europe, England and Wales has been the jurisdiction that has most closely followed the US in its race to incarcerate. By 2013, there were 10.2 million people across the world held in penal institutions; 2.4 million were in prison in the US. Russia (0.68 million), China (1.64 million) and the US together hold nearly half of the world's prisoners (Walmsley, 2015). The expansion of the use of imprisonment over the past 20 years has seen the increased privatisation of sections of the CJS. In Australia and the UK where privatisation has expanded rapidly, companies such as G4S have been given lucrative contracts to manage immigration detention centres and the electronic tagging of offenders. Wacquant (2009) shows the ways, in which, the 'prison industrial complex' has become a key factor in local employment, particularly in US rural areas. For employees, the prison provides secure, relatively well-paid jobs with benefits such as health insurance that are not widely available in generally impoverished communities. This creates a vicious circle where any reduction in the rate of imprisonment will be an economic threat, which contributes to political pressure at a local and national level.

In exploring these trends, it is important not to ignore wider cultural and social factors (Lacey, 2008). Liberal market economies with the concomitant deeply engrained individualism have become more punitive. Cavadino and Dignan (2006) in their analysis of penal policies and the use of imprisonment developed a political economy typology: neoliberal; conservative-corporatist; social democratic; and oriental corporatist. Examples of all these, apart from oriental corporatist, exist within Europe and the European Union. Germany and the Netherlands are notable as countries where the use of imprisonment has fallen. Subramanian and Shames (2013) show that this is due to policies such as the concentrated use of community penalties and suspended sentences in both countries. Downes and Hansen's (2006) analysis of 18 countries, including the UK and US, concluded that there was a clear relationship between welfare provision and penal policy: the lower the spending on welfare, the higher the rate of imprisonment.

Taylor (2003) argues that widely held views are 'not expressed in theoretical terms'. They are expressed in terms of images and stories. The importance of individual cases and media coverage cannot be underestimated in the areas of penal and mental health policy. In Chapter 3, the way that these very rare cases were used to construct a narrative of the failure of the policy was outlined. Similar themes emerge in the rise of the penal state. The increase in the use of imprisonment in the US and the UK has been driven by an often racialised image of the offender as a young, strong, physically fit male. The message is that such individuals pose a general threat to the wider populace. One of the most powerful of Hall et al's (2013) insights into the nature of state power is that violence and the need to respond to it generate a very strong support for its wider use by the state. Many commentators have made this link post 9/11, and Hall et al (2013) show that the early 1970s crises such as the UK response to Irish nationalist terrorism had similar impacts; for example, the targeting and demonising of minority communities and the introduction of legislation that restricted civil liberties. One potential role for social work as a profession is to challenge and counteract these narratives.

The Trencin Statement (WHO, 2008), which outlines the UN position on the treatment of prisoners, states that: 'Prisoners shall have access to the health services available in the country without discrimination on the grounds of their legal situation.'

The prison population is overwhelmingly drawn from the most marginalised communities. This is reflected in both the physical and mental health care of offenders. As the Royal College of Nursing (RCN) (2001) outlined, there is a higher incidence of long-term conditions and chronic disease among the offender population compared to the general population. These conditions include coronary heart disease, diabetes, mental health issues, substance misuse and HIV. Throughout the world, women are incarcerated at lower rates than men, but this is rising; since 2000 the global female prison population has risen by 50 per cent (Walmsley, 2015). This is largely explained by the gender differences in crime rates – women commit less crime than men. The Corston Inquiry (2007) was set up to look at the issues that arise from the imprisonment of women in England and Wales. The

Inquiry was established following a rise in cases of suicide and self-harm. Women are much less likely to commit violent or other serious offences than men, meaning that they are more likely to be sentenced to shorter periods in custody. The Corston Inquiry gives a stark outline of the wider factors in the lives of the women in custody: 37 per cent attempted suicide at some time in their life; 51 per cent have severe and enduring mental illness; over 50 per cent had been subjected to domestic abuse; and one in three had been sexually abused.

The expansion of the use of imprisonment has been most dramatic in the US. The result is a huge prison industrial complex (Gottschalk, 2006, Wacquant, 2009, Alexander, 2012). Simon (2014) terms this the 'arc of punitiveness', which began in the mid-1970s driven by populist responses to increases in violent crime and the politicisation of the law and order debate. The US is an outlier in this field, but the use of imprisonment has increased across Europe with England and Wales most closely following the US trends. Race is clearly an issue – it is not one that just applies in the US. In the UK, African-Caribbean citizens are imprisoned at a rate of 6.8 per 1,000 compared to 1.3 per 1,000 among white citizens. Of the UK prison population, 27 per cent comes from a BAME background and over two thirds of that group are serving sentences of over four years (1990 Trust, 2010). Berman (2012) reports that in June 2011 13.4 per cent of the prison population, where ethnicity was recorded, was black. The Lammy Review (2017) found that there had been no significant improvement. BAME citizens represent 14 per cent of the overall population in England and Wales but 25 per cent of the adult prison population. The situation is even more stark for young offenders where BAME individuals make up 41 per cent of those under 18 in custody.

The use of imprisonment is an issue that should be of concern to social work (Cummins, 2017). This is not simply because social workers will be working with individuals, families and communities who have experienced the impact of imprisonment. It should form part of a broader concern for human rights. Social work needs to question the use of imprisonment but also conditions in prison and issues such as access to healthcare. In writing the judgement in *Brown v. Plata,* Justice Kennedy concluded 'prisoners retain the essence of human dignity ... A prison that deprives prisoners of basic sustenance, including adequate medical care, is incompatible with the concept of human dignity and has no place in a civilized society.' The idea of dignity can be a starting point for the transformation of the CJS. The use of imprisonment, despite the manifest evidence of its failure, remains deeply entrenched in public policy.

In 1990, response to a previous crisis in the prison system in England and Wales led to prison riots, including one at Strangeways Prison in Manchester. The Strangeways riot was the longest in UK penal history and a public inquiry (Woolf, 1991) was conducted. The riots were a response to overcrowding and the poor conditions in prisons including the practice of 'slopping out' – where prisoners had to use a bucket as a toilet and empty them each morning. The practice was abolished in England in 1995. It should be noted that the prison population, at that time of the riots, was less than half what it is now. The Woolf Report (1991) was a blueprint for an improved prison system. The Home Office developed policies to reduce imprisonment on the basis that 'prison is an expensive way of making bad people worse'. These liberal moves were abandoned under subsequent governments committed to the idea that 'prison works' (Gottschalk, 2006). From that point onwards the prison population has continued to grow.

Mental disorder and offending

In this chapter, we are exploring the intersection between two very significant social policies: deinstitutionalisation, and the rise of the penal state. There are some contradictions between and within the policies explored. The general thrust of mental health policy has been to divert individuals from the CJS if possible (Cummins, 2006). This raises several fundamental questions about the prison and mental health policy but also broader ethical issues. The current difficulties in both prisons and mental health services illustrate that diversion, if it is achievable, requires robust and well-funded community mental services.

The term 'mentally disordered offender', at first glance, appears fairly straightforward. However, it has within it two fundamental questions: What is meant by *mental disorder*? Who do we deem an *offender*? These terms are used loosely as they cover such a wide range of huge behaviour. One common theme is that they create complex ethical and philosophical challenges. The bio-medical model does not fit easily into the mental health field (Eastman and Starling, 2006). It is a very powerful cultural trope that sees mental illness, particularly the most serious forms, as changing the character or personality of an individual. The existence and impact of mental illness has huge implications in the CJS field. The CJS has to address questions such as autonomy and responsibility in coming to decisions about guilt, culpability and sentencing. Therefore, psychiatric diagnosis has a role to play in the CJS. For example, the reform of the Mental Health Act

(2007) created the term 'dangerous and severe personality disorder'. This is a purely legal term. It was not developed in psychiatric discourse.

Autonomy

Autonomy is one of the key features of the Anglo-American legal tradition. It is assumed that individuals are free to act. If individuals are coerced in some way into committing an offence, they cannot be acting in an autonomous fashion. This approach has hugely important implications in this sphere. Nagel (1970) outlines a model of autonomy arguing that for behaviour to be viewed as intentional an individual must act on a belief or desire. He then adds another leg to the model: 'critical scrutiny'. The basis for the belief or desires must be rational. A decision based on an irrational belief will not pass this test. Therefore, the law should view these cases differently. This is a very significant standard and will not apply to most cases where individuals are regarded are mentally ill. The most high profile cases provide the most difficult challenges. For example, Hinckley's shooting of US President Ronald Reagan was the result of a delusional belief system in which not only did the President approved of his actions but also they would lead to Jodie Foster becoming his lover (Lipkin, 1990). These ideas cannot pass Nagel's test of critical scrutiny. This is clearly a rare and highly unusual example. However, it demonstrates the fundamental principles that need to be considered.

Punishment

The notion of autonomy is inextricably linked to punishment. Hence the importance of Nagel's notion of 'critical scrutiny'. The mental health systems and CJS overlap in complex ways. Punishment is based on the notion that the offender took a conscious, rational decision to ignore or break the law. They were not coerced. Thus, an offender can only be punished if they have willingly committed the offence. This is usually justified by reducing offending by both that individual and the wider deterrent effect. Offenders are viewed as moral agents who have chosen a particular course of action. Becker's (1968) influential Rational Choice Theory of offending is the clearest exposition of this approach.

Mental disorders potentially impact on thinking and decision making. A fundamental question is the extent, if any, that mental disorder can be said to lead directly to an offence. It should be emphasised that these are a very small minority of cases. Szmulker (2000) in his criticism of the community care inquiries of the 1980s and 1990s argues that these reports almost always deny that offenders have any choice or agency. Such symptoms can affect the individual's ability to act as a moral agent. Morse (2003) suggests that such accounts are inaccurate. He argues that a person experiencing hallucinations retains the ability to act intentionally, to act for reasons. Hinckley had clear reasons for acting. The issue for the CJS is to what extent the delusional basis of those reasons should be a mitigating factor.

Singleton et al's study (1998) is now over 20 years old but remains the benchmark study in the UK of the mental health needs of prisoners. Fazel and Seewald (2012) carried out a meta-analysis of studies of prisoners' mental health. Prisoners generally experience higher rates of mental illness than the general population, but these figures need to be approached with caution. Offenders are much more likely to have experienced a range of factors and life events that might contribute to or increase the possibility of adult mental health problems as adults. These would include experiencing poverty, being a victim of violent crime and sexual offences and being in the care of the local authority as a child (Marmot, 2010; Karban, 2016). Research has consistently highlighted the complex mental needs of prisoners. These occur alongside comorbidity of mental illness and substance misuse (Fazel et al, 2016; Bebbington, 2017; Bartlett and Hollins, 2018). These figures appear to have remained unchanged for over a decade. This research has also consistently demonstrated high rates of comorbidity between mental illness and substance misuse. This combination has profound health and social implications.

Fazel et al's (2012) study indicates that prisoners are a particularly at-risk group for suicide and self-harm. For male prisoners the rate is 3–6 times higher and for female prisoners the rate is 6 times higher than the wider community. It should be noted that the risk factors for self-harm and suicide, such as drug and substance misuse problems, experience of abuse and/or sexual violence, are all higher among men and women in prison. There are differential patterns identified here, including lower rates of suicide and self-harm among BAME prisoners.

Fazel et al (2012) also examine violence and victimisation. People with mental health problems are more likely than other groups in the general population to be subject to violence. Violence is almost taken as a given of daily prison life but there is little research that examines its prevalence. Studies indicate that physical assault is 13–27 times more common in prison than in the community (Fazel et al, 2017). The prison culture makes it difficult to carry out work in this area as assaults are likely to be under-reported, mostly because of the possible consequences of being seen as an informer. Fazel et al (2012) concluded that both male and female prisoners experiencing mental health problems were more vulnerable to sexual violence and physical assault.

Fazel et al (2012) argue that there is a need for a robust and systematic assessment of prisoners for mental health problems, alongside acute detox services on arrival at all prisons. Alongside these, there is the need for the provision of trauma-focused and gender specific interventions within the prison setting and the development of suicide prevention strategies, including monitoring and assessment of prisons and staff training. These recommendations are calling for the current best practice in community mental health to be applied to the prison setting.

Policing and mental illness

There has been an increasing focus on the role of the police in responding to the mental health crises. This has gone up the policy agenda. However, it is not a new issue and has appeared in various forms and configurations since the introduction of deinstitutionalisation. In Lipsky's classic *Street Level Bureaucracy* (2010), the term 'street level psychiatrist' was used to capture the role that the police, almost totally unwillingly, were being drawn into playing. One of the key features of Teplin's (1984) criminalisation of the mentally ill argument stems from the role of the police and increased police contact. In Teplin's (1984) seminal study of policing and mental illness, she used the term 'mercy booking' to describe the situation where the police arrest an individual because they felt that this would ensure that a vulnerable person was given food and shelter – even if it was in custody. Prior to this, Bittner (1967, 1970) had indicated that police beat officers were becoming increasingly involved in mental health work.

The role of the police was highlighted in several community care inquiries in the 1990s – most notably the Ritchie Inquiry (1994). In the modern context, there are concerns from the police that they are being increasingly called on because of the gaps in community mental health services. This is a role that police officers often feel ill equipped to undertake. The police role is thus a combination of preventing crime, detecting and apprehending those who have committed offences, and a more general one (Bittner 1967). This has always been the case since the establishment of the modern police force. However, the pressures have increased since the development of deinstitutionalisation and the policies of austerity adopted in the UK since 2010.

The recent retrenchment in mental health and wider public services mean that the police face increasing demands in this area (Cummins and Edmondson, 2016). Police involvement in mental health work has to be viewed as part of their role in wider community safety and the protection of vulnerable people. Wolff (2005) argues that the police have always had what might be termed a 'quasi social work' role. This is vital work, but mental health work does not fit easily with the aspects of 'cop culture' that Reiner (2000) identifies. For example, there is often not an immediate response in terms of action that can be taken. It is an area that does create challenges for police services (Carey, 2001; Lurigio and Watson, 2010). These challenges are both individual and organisational.

Wood et al's (2011) review of trends in the UK, Canada and the US concludes that the same issues arise across the countries: a combination of reduced psychiatric provision and poorly funded community services has led to increased pressure on police officers who often receive little or no specific mental health training. Police officers, particularly in urban areas, deal with incidents that relate in some way or another to mental illness on almost daily basis. Lord Adebowale (2013) concluded mental health is core police business. This should be taken to mean that dealing with individuals experiencing mental distress is a key feature of the working week of most police officers. This is a slightly different argument to the 'criminalisation of the mentally ill' argument. If one regards the role of the police as fundamentally a law and order one, then any police involvement could be used to support the criminalisation hypothesis.

The criminalisation of mental illness hypothesis

Teplin's (1984) study has been hugely influential. It showed that police officers were increasingly being drawn into mental health work. The study was one of the first to highlight that deinstitutionalisation was leading to people with mental health problems coming into increasing contact with the CJS. Bittner (1967a, 1967b, 1970) had previously drawn attention to this new trend. On the surface, these trends appear to offer support to the Penrose Hypothesis. It is important to recognise that there are always historical and national factors that apply. It is, therefore, not always possible to simple map developments from one jurisdiction on to another. However, the US experience does have a number of echoes of the development of community care in England and Wales – particularly in regard to the increased involvement of the police and other CJS professionals in the provision of some forms of mental health support.

The Bradley (2008) and Adebowale (2013) reports both highlighted concerns about the ways in which CJS professionals were being called on to respond to those in mental health crisis. The Corston Inquiry (2007), in calling for a new approach to the treatment of women in the CJS, focused very much on the mental health needs of this cohort. Seddon (2009) noted that this is a long standing perspective that sees female criminality, almost by definition, as evidence of some form of mental pathology. A series of reports from the Prisons Inspectorate (HMIP 2017; 2018) have emphasized that prison is not, and can never really be, a therapeutic institution. Despite this, in the UK at present, there is not the powerful anti-mass incarceration movement that exists in the US.

How can we explain the fact that people with mental health problems are increasingly drawn into the CJS? This is despite the fact that, in the UK, there is a history of official policy initiatives to divert people out of the CJS that is now nearly 30 years old (Cummins, 2006). The first thing to note is that there has been a series of shifts in broad social and welfare policy that are part of this picture. Wacquant (2010) proposes that what he terms 'prison fare' is an endogenous feature of neoliberal regimes; the Police, Courts and Prisons are key political institutions that not only manage the inequality and marginality, but are also active in its production and maintenance. 'Advanced marginality' is used to convey the ways that significant groups of people are effectively locked out of access to the resources and mechanisms of modern citizenship such as decent education, health, social care and full-time permanent, well-paid, employment. Although Wacquant's work has focused on the US, these trends can be identified across other advanced economies.

Those who argued for the closure of the asylums wanted them replaced with well-funded and resourced community centres. They were certainly not arguing that the state should have no role in mental health provision. However, this vision has never been realised. Deinstitutionalisation could be taken to refer to those former patients who were resettled into the community. The first wave of this process was largely positive (Leff and Triemann, 2000). However, the optimism began to fade. Poor community mental health and welfare services expose vulnerable individuals to a series of risks in addition to poor health. These risks include living in poor quality accommodation and homelessness. The rise in homelessness was one of the first signs that community care was struggling. Changes in policy such as laws on loitering in the States and anti-social behaviour orders in the UK lead to the greater surveillance of public spaces (Wacquant, 2009). These, in effect, criminalise homelessness and poverty (Barr, 2001 and Cummins, 2012). Teplin (1984) outlines the way that increases in police contact increase the likelihood that someone with a mental health problem will be arrested, possibly for a minor issue. Teplin (1984) identified what she termed 'mercy bookings' where concerned officers arrested an individual because they thought that this would mean that they could access some support or at least they would have a bed and food for a short period. Once in the CJS, people who have mental health problems then face a number of difficulties including access to appropriate treatment, and bullying and harassment.

The criminalisation hypothesis does not completely explain the way that the CJS has played an increasing role in the provision of mental health care. One has to be very careful in applying this conceptual tool. It is important to remember that the CJS is a complex and often confusing space such that it is doubtful whether it can actually be described as a system. There are so many points of contact and decision making. CJS professionals work in a range of settings and respond to a range of pressures and individual circumstances. The overwhelming majority of staff have no formal mental health training. In addition, the idea that people with mental health problems somehow form a distinctive group within the CJS or prison systems is false. The presentation of mental illness is not consistent. Finally, a person can be mentally ill and act knowingly in the commission of an offence. Acknowledging all of this, during the period of deinstitutionalisation and after, the failure to build adequate community mental health services and a more punitive approach to social policy generally led to vulnerable people with mental health problems being drawn into the CJS. It is likely that, for a combination of reasons, there will always be individuals with mental health problems in contact with CJS professionals. The aim should be to limit this as far as is possible.

Conclusion

The retrenchment of the welfare state clearly has the greatest impact on the most vulnerable and marginalised. These trends have been exacerbated by the policies of austerity. The *New York Times* reported that austerity had led to the retooling of the welfare state (Goodman, 2018). The result is a residual system that has more in common with the US system than it does with the social democratic and corporatist systems of Europe. In November 2018, the UN Rapporteur (Alston, 2018) reported that the UK is the fifth largest economy in the world but, as a result of austerity, 14 million people – one fifth of the population – are living in poverty. The impact of the development and life chances of children and young people is described as 'not just a disgrace but a social calamity and an economic disaster, all rolled into one' (Alston, 2018: 1).

The policy of deinstitutionalisation is followed across the world. At the same time, there has been a clear shift towards a more punitive prison policy. As Wacquant (2009) argues, throughout the industrialised world there has been a large prison building programme and investment in the CJS. Gunn (2000) and Kelly (2007) found that the reduction in the number of psychiatric beds in the UK occurred at the same time as the rise in the prison population, as Penrose predicted. The clash of the two policies outlined previously – deinstitutionalisation and mass incarceration – seems to provide evidence to support Penrose's original hypothesis. Large and Nielssen (2009) undertook a review of Penrose's original hypothesis using data from 158 countries. They suggest one of the main features of Penrose's argument is that there is an unchanging proportion of any population that will need, or be deemed to need, some form of institutional control. They concluded that though there was a positive correlation between prison and psychiatric populations in low and middle income countries, there was no such relationship in high income countries.

Penrose's hypothesis can be seen as a statistical argument, examining the relationship between two major institutions – prison custody and psychiatric care. There are a number of problems that arise here. Such an approach equates crime and mental illness. In addition, it fails to explore the reasons behind the changes in patterns of use of the two institutions. The increase in the use of prison continues despite the general reduction in the crime rate (Garland, 2001). Therefore, it is part of a wider change in society and government attitudes rather than simply a response to crime. The changes in the use of institutional psychiatric care are the result of a combination of social attitudes, improved medical and treatment approaches, recognition of the cost of inpatient treatment and recognition that citizens should not lose their civic and human rights because of mental ill-health.

Two of the key institutions of modernity are the asylum and the prison (Foucault, 2003; 2012). The representation of them as two distinct regimes – one punitive, the other therapeutic – provides a very limited analysis. It is based on the notion that there is some clear boundaries and a systemic way of allocating individuals to these institutions. It assumes that the asylum was a therapeutic regime and that no rehabilitation, in the broadest sense, occurs or has occurred in prisons. Both these positions are hugely debated. This is one of the key weaknesses of the position that Penrose puts forward. However, it is readily apparent that the decline of institutionalised psychiatric care occurred as the penal state expanded. As previously outlined, the relationship between these policies and their impact is complex and messy. Metzl (2010) argues that the changes reflect nature in both the approach to deviance and mental illness. Metzl (2010) outlines the way that in the post-civil rights period, the diagnosis of mental illness in the US underwent a huge shift. It moved from being a diagnosis associated with passivity, anxiety and social isolation to one associated with aggression, violence and a refusal to conform to social norms. During this period, the representative figure of this diagnosis moved from a white, often middle class, middle aged woman to a young, working class black man. As noted in the discussion of the media coverage of inquiries (in Chapter 3), the most high profile cases such as the Clunis case (Cummins, 2010) reproduced long standing racialised stereotypes of mental illness.

One of the consequences of the ongoing failures of community care has seen CJS professionals become more involved in responding to those in mental health crisis. The boundaries between the mental health system and the CJS appear more blurred and confusing than ever. The focus is not on clearly important philosophical debates about autonomy or responsibility and the nature of mens rea. There is a danger that 'mad' or 'bad' limits our understanding of the causality of offending while at the same stigmatising mental illness. There are some more practice and system focused issues that need to be considered – these include: the role of the police; how to provide appropriate mental health care in prisons; and how can we develop systems that respond more effectively to the needs of women in prison. The history of penal policy in the era of community care demonstrates that this will only be achieved by reducing the size of the prison population while at the same time investing in community mental health services. In effect, this is a modern version of Penrose, with a moral not a statistical argument.

6

Reform or revolution? Mental health legislation and the development of community care

Introduction

This chapter will explore the development of mental health legislation from the introduction of the 1983 Mental Health Act (MHA) to the introduction of Community Treatment Orders (CTOs) in the reforms of 2007. The chapter ends with a brief discussion of the Wessely review of the MHA that was completed in 2018. Reform of mental health legislation reflects two potentially conflicting strands. One is the state's power to incarcerate the 'mad', the other is the move to protect the civil rights of those who are subject to such legislation.

The development of legislation reflects the broader pattern of community care as a policy. The initial optimism and progressive reforms of the early 1980s are overtaken by a more managerialist, pragmatic approach which focuses on risk and risk management. As discussed in Chapter 3, high profile cases and the way that they were reported in the media had a significant influence on the way that these policies were framed. Frank Dobson famously said in 1998 that community care has failed (BBC News, 1998). This may be a sweeping generalisation. However, I think it is possible to argue that the introduction of CTOs marks the symbolic end of official commitment to community care.

Mental health legislation before the 1983 MHA

The development of mental health policy is messy, complex and at times somewhat contradictory. It reflects not only broader social, cultural and economic trends but the relative positions of professionals, the strength of campaigning and service user groups, responses to institutional scandals and developments in treatments. In addition, there has always been a role for individual social reformers, who have challenged abusive conditions and practices. Finally, it would be naive to overlook the fiscal pressures that play such a key role in the implementation of any social policy.

Scull (1986) notes that the development of mental health and other areas of policy such as those in the criminal field have involved a greater role for the modern state. Within this field, one sees the emergence of new fields and new professionals who claim expertise in the identification, assessment and treatment/management of conditions and individuals. Prior to the modern view of madness as a form of illness, there was little specific specialist provision for those regarded as mad (Foucault, 2003). Foucault (2003) controversially argues that the 'mad' were in a sense tolerated – treated as the village fool or expelled from their own parishes to wander the countryside. One of the key strands of his argument is that they were not institutionalised. This is a modern practice. There has always been and continues to be a divide between the experiences of the poor and the rich. Rich families were able to send their relatives to private madhouses or 'care' for them in their own homes. The Poor Law Act 1601 placed a duty to the old and the sick, including 'idiots and lunatics'. Outdoor relief was provided. If the poor were unable to work due to infirmity, they could be placed in workhouses.

One of the recurring themes in the modern mental health field is attempts to overcome stigma and segregation. Segregation is clearly a physical but also a socio-psychological phenomenon. The two aspects are interrelated. Segregation was most clearly manifest in the asylum regime. The beginning of segregation and the first wave of asylums are linked to the Enlightenment emphasis on rationality. The 18th century saw the development of a series of private madhouses. In a recurring theme in mental health policy scandals in the condition in these unregulated institutions led to a government Inquiry. The result was the 1774 The Act for Regulating Private Madhouses. This Act saw the introduction of a requirement for medical certification for insanity. These provisions did not apply to pauper lunatics. By the beginning of the 19th century, it is possible to see the emergence of a biological model of insanity – at the time based on the notion that it was the result of physical imbalances in the body. At the same time, Tuke's model of moral treatment argued that the physical environment had a key role to play in the management of the disordered mind.

The Victorian period saw the establishment of the asylum system that became the focus of such criticisms in the post Second World War period. The Poor Law Amendment Act 1834 was not specifically concerned with the treatment of the mentally ill. The indoor relief in the workhouses was designed specifically to act as a deterrent to those who might make a claim. As pauper lunatics were seen as an increasing burden in this system, more of them were sent to the asylums. The Lunatics Asylums Act 1845 made it mandatory for each borough and county to provide a publicly funded asylum. The development of Social Darwinism in the 1880s and 1890s saw political concerns with what was termed the 'residuum' (Stedman-Jones, 2014). These concerns have been echoed in more modern debates about poverty, welfare and the role of the state (Cummins, 2018). These include poorer sections of society having too many children, which is seen as leading to increased demands on welfare and charities. Alongside there was a belief that the strength of nation state and Empire would be undermined and weakened by the behaviour of the growing poor. The result was a widespread belief in and acceptance of the key tenets of eugenics and social hygiene. It was argued that society was producing too many 'imbeciles' or 'inadequates'. Public figures such as George Bernard Shaw and Winston Churchill shared these beliefs (Carey, 2012). The 1886 Idiots' Act introduced an official distinction between 'lunatics', 'idiots' and 'imbeciles'. As a result, there were a series of separate asylums for the 'mentally subnormal'. The 1890 Lunacy Act revised the process of admission. It also strengthened the inspection and reporting procedures. The 1913 Moral Deficiency Act classified 'mental subnormality' into three categories: idiot, imbecile and feeble minded. It also saw the creation of the category 'moral imbecile'.

Prior to the First World War, psychiatry and the asylum system were heavily influenced by these notions of social hygiene. The experiences of the Great War had a profound impact on these notions. Shell shock was experienced by soldiers from all social classes. Sufferers included members of the officer class so the cause could not be identified as inferior breeding or a lack of character and moral fibre. Freudian and psychoanalytic theories became more influential. The Tavistock clinic opened in 1920. A Royal Commission on Lunacy and Mental Disorder was established in 1924. The Mental Treatment Act 1930 saw 'asylum' replaced by 'mental hospital' and 'lunatic' by 'patient'. Asylum and lunatic, however, remained powerful terms in popular culture. The act established three categories of patient: certified, voluntary and temporary. Temporary was a certified category but lasted up to six months. This was the first time that patients could admit themselves on a voluntary basis.

The 1959 Mental Health Act

The development of what we can identify as the modern welfare state in the post Second World War period saw an increasing acceptance and support of state intervention in health and social welfare (Kynaston, 2008). These trends were apparent in a range of fields including mental health. The Macmillan Commission, which established the framework for the Mental Treatment Act 1930, made a clear statement that mental disorder was a medical illness like any other: 'There is no clear line of demarcation between mental and physical illness' (Royal Commission, 1926). The creation of the NHS in 1948 incorporated mental hospitals into the broader system. Significant changes in the provision of mental health treatments occurred in the post war period. In 1954 neuroleptics (major tranquillisers for the treatment of psychotic symptoms) were introduced in the UK. These drugs marked a shift in treatment but were also immensely problematic because of their potential side effects. The criticisms of the mental hospital system – both in terms of the physical conditions and the denial of civic rights – became more vocal during the 1940s and 1950s. The Percy Commission was established, and this led to the Mental Health Act 1959. Despite the broader currents of optimism about the potential for new forms of service provision, the 1959 MHA was very much focused on hospital admission. The 1959 MHA defined mental disorder as 'mental illness; arrest or incomplete development of mind; psychopathic disorder; and any other disorder or disability of mind'. The 1959 MHA abolished the distinction between psychiatric and general hospitals. It was something of a forerunner of community care policies. Sections 25, 26 and 29 outlined the criteria for formal admission. Social workers also took on the role of mental welfare officers working in the community but were also involved in the formal admissions process. A tribunal system was also established for patient appeals. The Royal Commission of 1926 had examined the possibility of abolishing the magistrate's role in the commitment process. However, it was not until the introduction of the 1959 MHA that this occurred. It was at this point that the responsibility for the assessment and detention of the mentally ill became solely that of mental health professionals.

The 1983 Mental Health Act

The Mental Health Act 1983 was introduced followed a period of campaigning by MIND, which at time was headed by an American civil rights lawyer, Larry Gostin. Following his period at MIND, he became General Secretary of the UK's National Council for Civil Liberties (NCCL). He was at the NCCL during the Miners' Strike (1984–85). The NCCL produced a report which was critical of both the police and the striking miners. Gostin left the NCCL in the aftermath of this report, which argued that the NCCL should remain politically neutral if it were to protect civil liberties. He is now a professor at Georgetown University in Washington DC, where he is also the director of the O'Neill Institute for National and Global Health Law and director of the WHO Collaborating Center on Public Health Law and Human Rights. Under Gostin's leadership, MIND took a campaigning rights-based approached to mental health issues – seeing the law as one of the key tools in ensuring that people with mental health problems were not subject to abuse.

By the 1970s, one of the periodic pressures to reform legislation that is such a feature of the history of mental health policy was beginning to develop. This was triggered by a range of factors. As always in this field, scandals and inquiries had a role to play. The poor care and treatment of people with mental health problems and learning difficulties had been highlighted by scandals at Ely Hospital (1969), Farleigh Hospital (1971) and Whitingham Hospital (1972) (Fennell, 2002). Barbara Robb had published *Sans Everything* (1967). This collection provided a devastating account of the appalling conditions in long-stay wards at seven hospitals. As well as describing dirty overcrowded wards, *Sans Everything* contained examples of staff treatment of patients, for example, verbal and physical abuse. The collection also highlighted the lack of dignity in standard practices such as a 'production line' for the bathing of patients. These concerns led to a shift away from the processes of detention to the conditions on wards. Both are, of course, fundamental issues of human rights. A state cannot detain an individual in accordance with a rights-based approach and do so in physical conditions that amount to a breach of those rights. The wider developments in the mental health field – such as concerns about controversial treatments such as psychosurgery and a focus on the civil rights of patients in the US (Fennell, 2002) – meant mental health came to be viewed much more within a civil rights framework. The abuses of psychiatry in the Soviet Union (Faraone, 1982) were seen by radical critics such as Szasz and Laing (Cummins, 2018) as emblematic of the discipline. Gostin's arrival at MIND was thus timely as the human rights law had yet to play the hugely significant role that it would do in the mental health field.

Gostin became a highly influential figure in academic and public life. He certainly had a profound impact on MIND. It is hard to imagine now that MIND had not employed a legal officer until the arrival of the former Fulbright Scholar, Gostin. Gostin's period at MIND certainly marked something of a departure. Hilton (2007) quotes a personal communication that she received from a reviewer of a paper she wrote about this period:

> Smythe and Gostin turned [things] upside down; they also recruited into the staff a number of aggressive anti-psychiatrists who had political connections with the Far Left. The traditional co-operative methods were replaced by confrontation. Before Gostin, MIND had never had a legal rights officer, but he established a dominant position within the organisation. Smythe, who was a weak character, took a back seat. Gostin was brilliant at manipulating the media so that whenever a mental health issue came up, their first call was always to him.

Gostin (2007) outlines the way that legal challenge became a key tool in MIND's armoury. He discusses several examples of this. In 1980 *A v the United Kingdom,* the challenge led to the government agreeing a small settlement with a patient at Broadmoor. Gostin (2007) recounts how he was asked to go and see the patient, Mr Clarke at Broadmoor. Clarke was being held in seclusion in appalling, insanitary conditions. Initially, the psychiatrist would not allow Gostin to even see Clarke. The case of Nigel Smith was another test case that MIND brought in the mid-1970s. This was another case based on the appalling conditions in which patients were held. The European Court held that these conditions were so poor that they could, in themselves, amount to a breach of Article 3 of the European Convention on Human Rights – 'No one shall be subjected to torture or to inhuman or degrading treatment or punishment.'

MIND played a key role in exposing the abuse of the use of electroconvulsive therapy (ECT). It found that ECT was being used often in breach of Royal College of Psychiatrists (RCP) guidelines. The use of ECT and the treatment of sex offenders by Dr Loucas at Broadmoor was also challenged by MIND. Loucas had given patients ECT without anaesthetic or muscle relaxant. He had also conducted a series of experiments where he gave hormone treatment to sex offenders. These experiments were conducted without any ethical oversight. The patients grew breasts (Gostin, 2007). In the case of *X v the United Kingdom*, the European Court held that restricted patients had been denied an independent judicial review of their detention. This was a breach of Article 5(4) of the European Convention Human Rights (ECHR). This case was before the incorporation of the provisions of the ECHR into UK law with the passing of the HRA (1998). The case originated with four patients at Broadmoor Hospital who had been there for decades. The patients had been admitted to Broadmoor having committed nonviolent crimes.

In the highly influential *A Human Condition,* Gostin set out MIND's proposals for reform of the 1959 MHA. The title of the work captures the underlying ethos and value position that MIND/Gostin adopted. Mental illness should be viewed in the same way as physical illness. Those who experience mental illness should not be deprived of the fundamental rights that all citizens should enjoy. Volume 1 focused on the system for admission and discharge, review tribunals and inpatient rights including consent to treatment. Volume 2 was concerned with the Butler Committee Report (1975) and the treatment of, in the language of the time, mentally abnormal offenders. As the anonymous correspondent shows, Gostin provided a radical challenge to the British psychiatric establishment. In discussing this period, Gostin (2007) notes the hostility to the main thrust of the arguments in *A Human Condition*. He quotes a *Times* article which concluded that public acceptance of changes in policies towards the mentally ill was dependent on maintaining confidence that any revised laws would allow for dangerous individuals to be 'locked up'.

In *A Human Condition,* Gostin argued that compulsory detention did not of and in itself allow for compulsory treatment. He therefore put forward a proposal that all treatment of a hospital 'resident' who is unable to or does not consent should be reviewed by an independent body. He called this proposed body the Committee on the Rights and Responsibilities of Staff and Residents of Psychiatric Hospitals (CORR). CORR would consider the views of all those involved – based on principles of dignity and the least restrictive principle for interventions (Hilton, 2007). MIND and others were particularly concerned by treatments such as ECT and the use of experimental drugs. *A Human Condition* is a key text in the development of a rights-based approach to mental health law reform. It thus has an influence in the development of community care – the logic of a rights-based approach is based on a fundamental questioning of the role of compulsory treatment and institutions.

The 1983 MHA is something of a departure because of its focus on the admission process and the new protections that were introduced. The law is only one aspect of the mental health policy landscape – an important one. The focus on this aspect can often obscure the relative importance of other areas. In addition, there is a strong tendency for such reforms to overpromise and under-deliver in the sense that they are presented as being the solution to a whole range of policy issues. The majority of these are unlike to be resolved by a change in legislation. Such issues are the result of complex system issues as well as organisational cultures. In the 1983 MHA, there are two poles of reform – the rights of the patient, alongside a concern for public safety. The introduction of public safety into these debates has been criticised for being based on stigmatised views of the mentally ill. The 1983 MHA sets some limits on the use of compulsory powers. The fact that these decisions were now to be made by mental health professionals was seen by Parliament as way of protecting the position of patients. Of course, I accept that many service users then and now had little confidence that mental health professionals were the people to protect their rights.

The 1983 MHA clarified the consent to treatment provisions, providing additional safeguards for patients detained under the MHA, in cases where they are treated against their will. The Mental Health Act Commission (MHAC) was established oversee the use of the MHA. The MHAC produced an annual report on such issues on trends in the use of the MHA and other related matters. This role has subsequently been taken on by the Care Quality Commission (CQC). The final change was the creation of the Approved Social Worker (ASW) role. The role of the ASW – one I undertook – was to provide a social perspective in the MHA assessment. This included not only ensuring that the views of the person being assessed were considered but also exploring all alternative and community-based options to a formal MHA admission. Section 117 MHA created a duty on Health and Social Services Authorities to provide aftercare for patients who have been subject to Section 3 and Section 37 MHA admissions. The 1983 MHA was not a key driver in shaping the development of community care. It created the legal framework in which the policy of community care was played out in the late 1980s and early 1990s. This is an important point. When New Labour introduced the *Modernising Mental Health Services* (Department of Health, 1998) policy document, it identified the legal framework as one of the key weaknesses in mental health policy. The document argued that the law had been drawn up in a period when hospital-based care was the key element of mental health services.

There had been shifts in the balance between the rights of patients and concerns about public safety. The Care Programme Approach Circular was to take effect from April 1991. It was described as the specialist form of care management for people with mental health problems. In 1993, Ben Silcock, a young man with a diagnosis of schizophrenia, climbed into the lions' enclosure at London Zoo and was severely injured. His case was covered in detail, particularly by the

Daily Mail (Cummins, 2012). The director of SANE, Marjorie Wallace, argued that the case showed that the pendulum in policy had swung too far in favour of patients' rights and away from families and carers. Wallace suggested that professionals were ignoring the concerns of parents and downplayed the impact of cannabis use on mental health. These themes chimed with the broader *Daily Mail* view of the ills of the modern world and their causes. The then Secretary of State, Virginia Bottomley, introduced a ten-point plan as a response to the public concern. A number of the ten points were policy restatements. However, they did include supervision registers – Mental Health Trusts were required to keep registers of people deemed to be a risk to others. If a patient moved, then the information was to be passed on to the Trust for their new address. This document included a proposal for a community treatment order. At the time, the RCP had already been lobbying for such a move. These proposals were eventually dropped as they were likely to breach the European Convention on Human Rights. The Mental Health (Patients in the Community) Act 1995, introduced a watered-down version of it. The provisions gave a named supervisor the power to convey a patient to hospital, but no power to detain them once there. It was therefore rarely used.

Supervised CTOs

The introduction of the CTO was the most significant of the 2007 MHA reforms. It can be imposed when a patient who has been detained under Section 3 is discharged from hospital. Conditions that can be placed on the discharge might include:

- having to live in a certain place;
- being tested for alcohol or illegal drugs;
- attending appointments for treatment.

The CTO introduced the power of recall to hospital if the responsible clinician has concerns that:

- the patient needs medical treatment in hospital for a mental disorder;
- there would be risk of harm to the health or safety of the patient or of others.

The power of recall means that a patient can be admitted to hospital for up to 72 hours. Decisions can be then made about future treatment plans and support.

CTOs were introduced by the 2007 reform of the MHA. However, looking back at the history of community care, the recommendation for the introduction of a CTO or similar legislation was a consistent feature of a number of mental health inquiries from the late 1980s/ early 1990s onwards. In particular, inquiries such as the Ritchie Inquiry into the care and treatment of Christopher Clunis concluded that such a change would allow services to intervene at a much earlier stage. The period of deinstitutionalisation saw the introduction some form of compulsory community treatment in several jurisdictions (Lawton-Smith and Dawson, 2008). Vergunst et al (2017) found that CTOs of one form or another exist in over 70 mental health systems across North America, Europe and Australasia. Those in favour of the CTOs argue that their use puts pressure on services to ensure that they provide adequate community mental health services to support individuals. It should be noted that an individual has to be subject to Section 3 of the Mental Health Act for a CTO to be considered, so mental health services have an ongoing duty under Section 117 MHA to provide aftercare. In theory, CTOs should avoid repeated admissions to hospital. The Mental Health (Patients in the Community) Act 1995 introduced supervised discharge, which can be viewed as a forerunner of the legislation that was finally introduced. The major difference between the two pieces of legislation was that supervised discharge did not include any powers of recall. If a patient did not comply with the conditions or there were concerns about their mental health, then professionals would have to arrange a further MHA assessment. The CTOs removed this requirement and the protections that these processes afford to patients. The CTOs represent a significant shift in the balance between patients and the wider society.

The case for the introduction of the CTO is a straightforward one. It will prevent repeated admissions to hospital and the distress and disruption that this entails. The focus in the legislation and the debates surrounding it is on one aspect of treatment – medication. The argument is that service users may become unwell or experience a relapse because the they fail to take medication (Department of Health, 2006). Maden (2007) has estimated that generally compliance rates are often under 50 per cent in circumstances where people experience chronic conditions. Despite a whole series of moves and policies that seek to place physical and mental health on similar footing, the area of consent remains a key difference. In the case of treatment for physical health care, doctors can only act with the informed consent of the patient. If an individual has capacity, then they can decide whether to accept or refuse the treatment. Szmukler (2018) argues that this key difference in the area of mental health law means that is it fundamentally discriminatory and stigmatising.

The introduction of CTOs was a response to concerns about the failings of community mental health services but also part of broader patterns in social welfare policy (Cummins, 2012). These broader patterns are a shift to a focus on risk and risk management. There are clearly a series of risks that arise in the mental health field. The first is the potential for the development of a mental health problem. These risks are not distributed evenly (Marmot, 2010; Karban, 2016). There then follows a series of risks linked to the experience of mental health problems – these include symptoms but also the wider social impacts such as stigma. In discussing risk, the levels of potential personal distress (Scull, 1989) are often overlooked or minimised. In addition, one needs to acknowledge the risk of serious harm to individuals or others. The most serious concern is the risk of death as a result of mental illness, either to the individual or someone else. The links between mental state and these outcomes are complex and not straightforward. The National Suicide Prevention Strategy in England and Wales suggested that 200 suicides per year were linked with followed non-compliance (National Institute for Mental Health in England, 2007). As was noted in Chapter 3, the media representation of community care created the impression that there had been an increase in homicides committed by people experiencing mental health problems. This was a very powerful view despite the fact that there had been no real increase in the number of such homicides (Taylor and Gunn, 1999). The Department of Health stated that there were around 50 such homicides per year in England and Wales. Large et al's 2008 study indicated that the number was less than 20 per year. This is not to deny or minimise the catastrophic impact of such events. It is rather to put them in a context and ask profound questions about the role that mental health services specifically can have in prevention.

Non-compliance with medication is presented as a key, if not *the* key, feature of relapse. Relapse in this model is thus a purely medical phenomenon and social factors and pressures are simply taken as a given or ignored. Non-compliance – an interesting term in itself as it is not one that is generally used in other areas of medicine – is seen as an indicator that the patient lacks insight. Insight is something of a vague term, but it includes an awareness of illness but also the benefits of prescribed treatment. The point here is that not taking medication is never a presented as a positive choice or a decision that may be based on rational factors, for example, deciding not to take medication because of potential side effects. Lack of insight is seen as a potential feature of serious psychotic illness and of non-compliance (Farnham and James, 2000). Amador (2006) goes further and suggests that this lack of insight is a permanent feature of conditions such as schizophrenia. This, of course, implies that no decision could be seen as rational. Thus, CTOs are presented as a necessary, paternalistic feature that is required to manage risk.

The arguments that were put forward for the introduction of CTOs were a mixture of the paternalistic – this will lead to less disruption in the lives of service users – and the utilitarian – it is necessary to restrict the liberty of a small group of individuals to protect the wider public. Szmukler (2018) argues that this not only overrides the liberty claims of an already marginalised group but also is based on an assumption about the predictably of violence. In addition, these models assume that the causal links between mental illness and violence are clear (Szmukler, 2018). Alongside this strand of analysis, there is a Foucauldian perspective that focuses on psychiatry as a site of the exercise of power relations (Foucault, 2003). One of the fundamental criticisms of Foucault's analysis is that it ignores or denies the agency of individuals, seeing them as helpless within the power structures of the mental health system (Scull, 1989; Giddens, 1991; Fendler, 2004). The claim that Foucault presents individuals as passive is one that is disputed (Stone, 1982). Individuals have and exercise agency – there would be no debates about compulsory treatment orders if they did not do so. Non-compliance can be constructed as a form of resistance (Chambers, 2005). The use of language is significant here. Terms such as resistance have their roots in an explicitly political discourse.

Any consideration of these issues must examine structural issues but also individual circumstances. The history of mental health services has been one of exclusion and marginalisation – 'the silencing of voices'. One of the most profound of Foucault's (2003) insights is that social, cultural economic and political factors determine how 'madness' is constructed and experienced within a society. In analysing this experience, we need to explore below the surface of a society to examine to explore these intellectual and cultural currents. Thus, the late 1980s and 1990s can be seen as a period where these currents moved towards a more risk and managerial orientated focus. These moves involved a particular social construction of the 'psychiatric patient', one that emphasised dangers and risk of violence. This then becomes a driver of mental health policy – for all. Barnes et al (2006) found that people working with mental health service users had difficulty in being heard. The views of those who had been compulsorily treated were often marginalised. Banongo et al's (2005) work on the experience of mental health forensic service users highlighted the way that service user perspectives were discounted or ignored. Service users saw services as focused on paperwork and tick box approaches to manage risk. This is a criticism that has been applied across all mental health systems not just forensic ones (Cummins, 2018).

One of the key arguments for CTOs is that they reduce the number of readmissions and thus improve the quality of life of those who are subject to them. There is a secondary argument that the use of CTOs will ensure that patients receive aftercare. It should be noted here that patients must have been admitted under Section 3 to be made subject to a CTO on discharge. They are therefore entitled to aftercare under Section 117 MHA. This has been the case since the introduction of the 1983 MHA. The guarantee of aftercare argument thus amounts to saying that the loss of liberty will ensure that health and social welfare agencies will meet their statutory duties. The CTO in England and Wales is based on similar legislation that existed in New Zealand. Dawson and Romans (2001) found the CTO had a positive impact on a group of 'long-term patients' who were supported in the community for more than a year without readmission.

Since the initial proposals for the introduction of CTOs, there have been ethical objections to the legislation. Despite these concerns and the wider pressures on services that have made the use of the recall to hospital power difficult, if not impossible, in some areas, the use of the CTOs continues to grow. Focus in the research field has tended to measure their impact in terms of clinical symptoms. This can be viewed as a proxy measure for compliance. The research has also examined these impacts within a relatively short period – 12 months. This reflects a much broader trend within mental health research which has often pushed the day to day experiences of service users to the margins. Reducing the distress that serious mental illness causes is an aim that I assume we would all support. However, it is important to recognise that this distress is not simply about symptomatology, it is rooted in the daily lives and experiences of service users. This requires that the evaluation of any policy needs to consider broader measures such as social outcomes.

Vergunst et al (2017) collected data from 114 people subject to CTOs. This was part of the broader Oxford Community Treatment Order Evaluation Trial (OCTET) trial. The study explored the links between the CTO and the individual's social situation. In the cohort of 114: 76 (67 per cent) were male; 56 (49 per cent) were white British; 37 (33 per cent) were black; 15 (13 per cent) were Asian; 6

(5 per cent) were 'Mixed/Other'. 99 per cent were unemployed. The overwhelming majority of those in this study had been diagnosed with a psychotic disorder and had been unwell, on average, for a period for 15 years. In summary then, this would seem to be representative of the cohort of patients that the CTO was designed for. This study used a range of tools to get a detailed picture of the individual circumstances, including: Social Network Schedule; Objective Social Outcomes Index – gathers information about an individual's living situation; Euro-Qol – a self-completed questionnaire that assesses health related quality of life; Oxford Capability Questionnaire for Mental Health; and the Brief Psychiatric Rating Scale. Overall, the study concluded that CTO duration was not associated with any of the outcomes that were assessed – to put it another way, the CTO had no impact on social outcomes.

Coercion and the use of the MHA remains very largely under researched. The focus in debates about the reform of the MHA is often conducted at an abstract level. In these discussions, the experiences of service users (and their families and carers) is often marginalised. Vergunst et al's study concludes that CTOs do not offer, in practice, the long-term benefits that were claimed when they were introduced. On a practical level, the increased pressure on beds means that one of the key features of the CTO (the power of recall to hospital) has become more difficult to exercise.

This study demonstrates that across a range of very important measures the CTO was not associated with significantly improved outcomes. All of this begs the question: can the continued use of the CTO be justified? Vergunst et al's (2017) work provides a powerful argument against CTOs. It emphasises again the need in mental health research to take a much broader and longer view of the impact of coercive interventions.

The 2007 reforms also created the role of the Approved Mental Health Professional (AMHP). The duties and powers of the AMHP are virtually the same as the ASW. However, the role was opened to other professionals – community psychiatric nurses and psychologists, for example. The rationale for this was never that clear. There was certainly not a clamour for other professionals to take on this demanding and complex role. This might seem like a very technical or minor change. However, I would argue that it is symbolic of the marginalisation of the social aspects of mental health. The most important aspect of the ASW role was the bringing of a social dimension to the assessment. This is not to say that other professionals are not aware of such issues. It is, rather, to highlight the potential conflicts of interest that arise. If the

AMHP comes from a nursing background, then all three professionals involved in an assessment will be from a mental health background.

Morriss (2016a, 2016b) in her study of mental health social workers working as AMHPs in Community Mental Health Teams (CMHTs) found that social work faced a battle to establish a distinct professional identity. Morriss (2016b) shows that the relatively recent configuration of CMHT and Mental Health Trusts made this process more difficult. Social workers were recorded as feeling professionally isolated in an environment dominated by medical professionals and with a clinical ethos. These trends have been hardened by the focus on risk and risk management (Turner and Columbo, 2008; Cummins, 2018). In Morriss' (2016a) study, welfare work – such as dealing with housing and negotiating with other bureaucracies – was not held in the same regard as AMHP work. AMHP work was held in much higher prestige and seen to confer a level of professional regard. This is the result of the further training, the complex range of skills required to become an AMHP and the significance of the decisions that they make. There is an irony here: the work that is the bedrock of community mental health work had a lower status with professionals than the exercise of powers under the MHA.

Mental health law

There is an assumption that there is a consistent tension in the development of mental health law and policy. This tension is identified as being one between the rights of the individual and the rights of the wider community to protection. It should be noted that this discourse seems to be based on an acceptance of the notion that people with mental health problems will pose some sort of threat to the wider community. The broader discourse of human rights developed in the shadow of the atrocities and oppression of Nazism (Habermas, 2010). As discussed in Chapter 3, the image of the asylum as a concentration camp was a powerful image in the calls for reform. The UN Declaration of Human Rights states in Article 1 that 'All human beings are born free and equal in dignity and rights' (United Nations General Assembly, 1948). Abuses of human rights involve violations of human dignity. The protection of human rights is, therefore, based on calls to a set of moral values that we share. This discourse of human rights is based on notions of dignity. This modern notion is a recasting of Kant's (1996) categorical imperative that every person should be viewed as an 'end in themselves'. This approach contrasts with utilitarianism and other forms of consequentialism. The modern notion of dignity is contrasted by Habermas (2010) with the development of the liberal rights of freedom of association and religion and protections against arbitrary arrest.

The enjoyment of these classic democratic rights was seen as providing protections against the potential intrusion of the state into the private sphere of family life. It should be noted that these rights were not enjoyed by everyone or all groups. Women, ethnic minorities and people with mental health problems who were institutionalised are clear examples of groups who were denied the full rights of citizenship. The abuse that occurred in these settings and the examples that Gostin (2007) quotes are clearly violations of human dignity and the bodily integrity of individuals. Rawls (1971) suggests that liberal, political rights can only be fully enjoyed if they are accompanied by social, economic and cultural rights. The asylum system prevented this. Dworkin (1995) notes that dignity is both a powerful but also a vague concept.

Gostin and mental health: a human rights approach

Gostin (2007, 2012) argues that a human rights approach provides an important perspective in the mental health sphere. Human rights law allows for international monitoring of mental health policies and practices of a country. As noted in the previous section, individuals possess these rights because of their humanity. They are intertwined. There are three important areas where the notion of human rights is of particular value:

- *Admission and detention:* All legal systems allow for the detention of people with mental health problems with a view to treatment. States normally only detain in custody those who are suspected or have been found guilty of criminal offences. There is a need for a fundamental fairness in the process of compulsory admission. Civil confinement can be justified provided that its aim is to prevent future harm to the individual and that it is limited for as short a period as possible. Article 5 of the HRA – the right to liberty – allows for 'the lawful detention of persons for the prevention of the spread of infectious diseases, of persons of unsound mind, alcoholics or drug addicts, or vagrants'. Article 5(4) states that 'Everyone who is deprived of his liberty by arrest or detention shall be entitled to take proceedings by which the lawfulness of his detention shall be decided speedily by a court and his release ordered if the detention is not lawful'. Thus any decision to use compulsory power has to be based on a medical assessment. This was confirmed in the case of *Winterwerp v the Netherlands* decided in the EC. In reaching this decision, the EC held that:

- – Except in emergency cases, the decision must be based on objective medical expertise that the person is of 'unsound mind'.
- – The mental disorder must be of a kind or degree such that compulsory detention is required.
- – The patient can only be detained as long as the disorder persists.
- – Detention must be carried out following a legally prescribed process.

• *Inpatient conditions:* As noted, poor physical conditions or the use of treatments in a fashion that breaches standard medical ethics could amount to a breach of Article 3 of the HRA as it would be inhumane and degrading treatment.

• *Wider rights of citizenship:* The fact that an individual has mental health problems or has been admitted to hospital on a compulsory or voluntary basis should not mean they are denied wider rights of citizenship. This would include rights to association. The Equality Act (2010) makes much of the discrimination in employment that individuals faced illegal. Gostin (2012) gives example of cases that MIND brought to court where individuals had been dismissed purely because they experienced mental health problems.

Gostin (2007, 2012) has termed this broader approach to human rights and healthcare – including mental health care – the 'ideology of entitlement'. This approach uses the language of rights to argue that the powers of compulsory treatment should be limited, curtail professional power, improve the overall quality of mental health services and maintain the social and legal status of those who experience mental illness. Hoggett (1984) noted that the 1983 MHA was mainly constructed on the basis of pragmatic rather than principled arguments. She highlighted that there is a 'deep divide' in the legal oversight of mental health services. There is clearly the potential for effective legal intervention in the admission process and treatment in hospital. There is less potential for such oversight in community settings. Eastman (1994) argued that the MHA was actually underused, meaning that there was a shift in the civil rights/public protection balance that had not been intended. Laing (2000), in discussing the development of the MHA, notes that the 1983 MHA created a series of largely *negative* rights – for example, the tribunal system. There were few substantive rights or entitlements to services which would be regarded as *positive* ones. The provisions of Section 117 MHA and the entitlement to aftercare could be construed as a positive right. However, it applied to a relatively small, but increasing, group of patients. In addition, it was only applicable if a patient had been detained – if they had experienced a loss of liberty. Finally, one would have to question the effectiveness of the implementation of this right to aftercare in many cases.

Gostin's tenure at MIND saw him become a highly influential public figure. The profile of MIND was also raised. Rose (1985) argued that this focus on a rights-based approach is a limiting one. Rose highlights the *medicalisation of life* – the way that the causes and solutions to social and individual problems are seen as having psychological causes. This has increased the role of the *psy* professions. It also has had the tendency to individualise the causes. Rose (1985) argues that the widening of the influence of psy professions is based on contractual therapist/patient relationships. The focus here is on building relationships and positively seeking help. There are elements of this in mental health systems, but the shadow of compulsion looms large. Rose (1985) suggests that there is a fundamental rift between legalism or rights-based approaches and psychiatric discourse. Legalism is based on the application of rationality and a set of rules. This does not rule out discretion because this is present in all systems. Psychiatric discourse is much more ambiguous because of the nature of mental illness but also because of the individual nature of assessment.

Gostin (2007, 2012) acknowledges that the application of entitlement theory requires a level of social investment. This is one of the fundamental fault lines in the development of community care. It is important to emphasise that this is not simply about investment in mental health services. It is, rather, a recognition that poverty, inequality, racism and other forms of discrimination and oppression can have an impact on the development and prognosis on mental health problems (Marmot, 2010; Karban, 2016). In its most radical form, this argument sees psychiatry as a form of social control or an adjunct to the maintenance of late modern capitalism (Cummins, 2018). One of the most striking developments during the period of community care is that there has been an increase in the use of compulsory admission. Rose (1985) suggests that prior to the 1983 MHA compulsory powers were used in one in ten cases. This assumes that all voluntary admissions are genuinely voluntary, which I think is very much open to debate. Rose sees the increase in the use of the MHA as a failing. However, it is possible to argue that the use of compulsory powers at least creates a framework for the protection of patients that does not exist in voluntary cases. The developments discussed in this chapter highlight the contradictory nature of MHA law and policy. The establishment of safeguards and protections around the assessment and admission process in the 1983 MHA did not place community care on a strong footing. One clear lesson here is the inability of a rights-based approach to deliver resources. However, those who make this criticism of the rights-based approach have failed, to my mind, to outline a strategy that can or does guarantees social investment.

At the heart of the rights-based arguments for community care is an argument about the nature of citizenship and the relationship between the individual, the state and the wider community. If we accept that there should be occasions when the state can intervene in the lives of those experiencing mental illness, then we need to ensure that this is done only in the most limited cases. The creation of such compulsory powers also requires a system that allows for their use to be effectively challenged. Finally, it requires that the conditions in which people are detained do not breach human rights standards. The push towards deinstitutionalisation in the early 1960s was, in part, based on the recognition that the mental health system of the period failed this test. Somers (2008) argues that citizenship should not be viewed as simply a matter of formal legal rights. It requires the creation of a series of processes – legal, political and social. This combination ensures that citizens are or can be active members of a range of social and political communities. If such processes do not exist or are weak, then there is a gap between a formal declaration of rights and translating them into meaningful substantive rights in practice. Somers (2008), in her discussion of modern citizenship, uses the term from Arendt (1973) – the 'right to rights'. The existence of de jure rights does not mean that citizens can de facto enjoy them. This requires the membership of a polity Using this model, asylum patients of the 1950s and 1960s did not enjoy the rights of full citizenship. Somers (2008: 118) concludes that market fundamentalism has led to increasing numbers of people losing any meaningful membership of civil society. Citizenship has become contractualised and commodified. The beginning of these developments can be seen in the early 1980s.

Conclusion

Gostin (2007) sees the 1959 MHA and the 1983 MHA as moves towards a rights-based approach. The focus was, thus, inevitably concerned with the key areas of admission and treatment, and the 2007 reform marks a shift away from this. The review of the MHA was led by Genevera Richardson, a law professor from Kings's College London. The opposition to the initial reforms suggested by the Richardson Committee and other political factors meant that it took nearly ten years for the legislation to be enacted. However, the New Labour case for reform was made in *Modernising Mental Health Services* (Department of Health, 1998). This document outlined the structural and organisational factors that had led to the failings of community care. These included organisational and funding issues as well as a lack of support for families and carers. The document argued that the law was focused on an institutionalised model of care – admission and treatment. The argument was that this legislation could not cope with the new environment and demands of community care. There is an implicit assumption here that community care requires powers for community treatment. This argument is never explicitly made. It appears a rather weak one in my view. The reforms that New Labour introduced have to be linked to its wider view of citizenship. The 2007 reform is a significant move to a 'responsibility agenda'. The publication of *Modernising Mental Health Services* (Department of Health, 1998) is a hugely significant moment in mental health policy. Warden (1998) argued that it marked the end of community care. The use of the term in a positive sense was increasingly limited from the late 1980s onwards. It is now virtually non-existent. It is clear that the document marks the end of an official commitment to the idealism that underpinned community care. The pendulum had swung back towards concerns with public safety. In the process, the rights of individuals were significantly harmed. Recall to hospital without any requirement for a further formal mental health assessment represents a significant shift in the balance between individuals and the state. The fact that these reforms were passed with little or no opposition from libertarian politicians committed to the rights of individuals says a great deal about the status of those detained under the MHA.

When she arrived in Downing Street, Theresa May made a speech in which she outlined what she described as the 'burning injustices' in modern Britain. Mental health services and the overuse of the MHA was one of the areas she highlighted. This was a shock as many pointed out that she had been a senior figure in governments committed to austerity policies that had had a devastating impact on mental health services and the mental health of individuals (Cummins, 2018b). This was the architect of the so-called 'hostile environment' highlighting race and mental health services as an area of concern. The review was chaired by an eminent psychiatrist Professor Sir Simon Wessely and completed in December 2018 (Department of Health and Social Care, 2018).

In his foreword to the final report, Simon Wessely outlines the case for change. These concerns have echoes of earlier reviews that led to changes in legislation. Alongside the increase in the number of detentions, the review sought to address long standing concerns about the processes of admission under the MHA and patients' experiences on inpatient units. The review reports that there were 49,551 detentions under the MHA in 2017/18, excluding short-term orders such as Section 5(2) (Department of Health and Social Care, 2018: 44). There was a 40 per cent increase in detentions from 2005/06 to 2015/16. The risks of black patients, particularly young men, to be subject to CTOs were also noted. Black people were eight times more likely to be subject to a CTO than their white fellow citizens. These are trends that have been in existence for some time. The review proposes several significant changes to the MHA. It starts from the position that we need to move to an approach that is fundamentally rights-based. The key principles of the new MHA will be: choice and autonomy; least restriction; therapeutic benefit; and the person as an individual. These appear to be principles that few if any of us would not be able to accept. The previous history of mental health legislation demonstrates that, without wider social investment and a commitment to organisational and cultural change, such principles can become tokens rather than the drivers of real reform.

7

International perspectives

Introduction

This chapter will examine deinstitutionalisation in Italy, the United States and post-apartheid South Africa. In examining the different drivers and outcomes of policies in these areas, similar themes to the UK experience emerge. These include: the role of scandals in the pressure for change; the role of fiscal considerations in the development of policy; an initial period of optimism; and the impact of scandals. In Italy, the work of the psychiatrist Franco Basaglia was seen as a possible blueprint for wider reforms. Basaglia's work became very influential among radicals and the anti-psychiatry movement (Cummins, 2017). The US was at the forefront of the deinstitutionalisation policy. The links between the closure of psychiatric facilities and the expansion of the use of imprisonment have been most closely examined in this context. Finally, the chapter examines the total policy failure that led to the deaths of 144 patients in Gauteng Province, South Africa in 2014.

Basaglia: a psychiatric revolutionary

Franco Basaglia was a political radical, influenced by his own experiences in wartime Italy and the critical Marxist thinker, Antonio Gramsci. He argued that psychiatry and the treatment of the mentally ill could not be divorced from the wider social and political context, in which, it took place. As a radical critic of capitalism, he viewed the treatment of the mentally ill as an issue of social justice but also indicative of wider social injustices and inequalities. The values of mental health services thus reflect the wider values of the society. Basaglia concluded that institutionalised psychiatric care was inevitably abusive and would lead to the social isolation. He was clear that the asylum regime could not be reformed but would have to be abolished. For Basaglia, the revolution in psychiatric care required a huge shift from exclusion and isolation to inclusion and the establishment of humanitarian principles. He saw the institutionalised delivery of mental health care as representative of wider oppression. A challenge to it would be part of a wider challenge to social injustice. Basaglia saw his work as part of a potential wider progressive coalition. At the core of Basaglia's approach is a belief in the essential political nature of the structure and delivery of mental health care.

Foot's (2015) outstanding biography of Basaglia places his work and the psychiatric reforms he initiated in the context of post-war Italian politics. Basaglia was born in Venice in 1924. In 1944, he was arrested and imprisoned for his role in opposing local fascists. This was a key moment of his political and intellectual life. As is outlined in the next paragraph, Basaglia frequently compared the conditions that he experienced in prison to others that patients endured at the psychiatric hospital in Gorizia where Basaglia's radical reforms of Italian psychiatry services are best understood in the broader context of a radical political tradition. Basaglia was clearly influenced by the Italian political activist and philosopher, Antonio Gramsci (1891–1937). Gramsci emphasised the need to achieve what he termed hegemony. The concept of hegemony can be understood as the processes by which the dominant social class ensure that its moral, political and cultural values become the most powerful in society.

Basaglia's work is best understood within the context of the radical politics of 1968 (Cummins, 2018). Basaglia starts from a position that views the treatment of the mentally ill as an issue of rights. Institutions were abusive not simply because of the physical conditions but also because they meant that individuals who were mentally ill were being denied full citizenship. The physical conditions were a manifestation of capitalist values that focus on productivity – this group was seen as unproductive. In parallel processes, other marginalised groups were denied the enjoyment of full civic rights on the basis of their race, gender or sexual orientation.

Basaglia appeared destined for a glittering academic career but fell foul of institutional politics (Foot, 2015). As a result, he became director of a psychiatric clinic in Gorizia, a small town in Northern Italy on the border with modern day Slovenia. Basaglia's term in Gorizia might have been viewed as a period of exile or even banishment. It would have been viewed that way at the time. The geographical and professional isolation did not signal the end of his career and influence – it was the start of a remarkable rise. The move to Gorizia was the start of a revolution in Italian psychiatry, the influence of which was felt across Europe in the late 1970s and early 1980s.

When Basaglia arrived at the Gorizia asylum, the isolation of the institution had contributed to the development of a culture of neglect and abuse. The wards were in awful, often insanitary, conditions. Patients were physically restrained and violently assaulted. There are echoes here of other scandals and exposes that had played a key role in the criticisms of the asylum regime. Basaglia compared the conditions to those that he had experienced in prison. Primo Levy (the Holocaust survivor) and his accounts of his survival of Auschwitz were a profound influence on Basaglia. The psychiatrist made an explicit comparison between the two institutions – concentration camp and asylum. He argued that the asylum inmates as political refugees whose treatment exposed the fundamentally brutal and inhumane nature of capitalist society. A series of photographs by Raymond Depardon records the dehumanising conditions that Basaglia was committed to ending (see Howard, 2018).

It would be wrong to present Basaglia as a reformer. He was very much of the view that the asylum could not be reformed: it had to be abolished. It was an institution, representative of a morally and ethically corrupt system. He concluded that a revolution was required. Goffman's *Asylums* and the concept of a total institution was a key influence on Basaglia (Foot, 2015). A key focus of the changes introduced was attempts to create a different culture. The divide between patients and staff was, as far as possible, abolished. Significant elements of the coercive regime based on restraint were to be replaced by a relational approach. ECT had a totemic status of the abusive nature of modern institutionalised psychiatry. Its use was abolished. Instead of the previous system of ward rounds and groups of staff discussing patients, a series of open meetings were introduced. In these meetings, patients and staff debated issues before coming to a decision on major issues. Basaglia published a collection *L'Istituzione Negata (The Institution Denied)* which outlined the work at Gorizia and was widely read. In addition, a TV documentary Sergio Zavoli's *The Gardens of Abel* was shown in Italy in 1969. Zavoli, a left-wing Catholic, was broadly sympathetic to the thrust of the reforms and the film reflects this. As Foot (2015) notes events at Gorizia reflected the broader political movement of 1968 at its best and worst. The radical shift in attitudes, which included the recognition of the fundamental human dignity of those incarcerated in the asylum, the removal of many of the casual brutalities and indignities of daily life and a focus on relationship building, all stem from the anti-authoritarianism of the 1968 protests.

Basaglia's Law: Law 180

The Italian Mental Health Act of 1978 came to be known as Basaglia's Law or Law 180. It can be viewed as the culmination of Basaglia's work.

Its aim was to prevent the indefinite detention of vulnerable individuals. Law 180 removed dangerousness as a criterion for compulsory admission. The new criterion was that there was a therapeutic emergency. In addition, such admissions would be to a psychiatric unit in a general hospital. Law 180 abolished asylums. Prior to this, patients were in effect detained indefinitely. The regime that so appalled Basaglia meant that there was no realistic prospect of rehabilitation. Patients were trapped in corrosive and antitherapeutic systems. The asylums were to be abolished and replaced by community services and psychiatric wards in general hospitals or outpatient clinics. The Italian experience was frequently quoted by proponents of community care as a success and a potential model for service development. *Critical Psychiatry* (Ingleby, 1980), an influential text in the development of community care in the UK, has a chapter written by Basaglia outlining the reforms in Gorizia.

Basaglia's work has been the subject of much debate. As with the introduction of community care in other areas, it has been criticised for being utopian. Basaglia's opponents argued that the reforms did not adequately replace the asylum. The result, it is suggested, was to abandon some of the most vulnerable people. There are also echoes of the experience of community care in England and Wales: damage was done to public opinion of the reforms by violent crimes committed by patients or former patients (Cummins, 2010). Giovanni Miklus, on day release from Gorizia in 1968, killed his wife with a hammer. Basaglia and one of his colleagues were accused of manslaughter, although both were eventually cleared. In February 1972, Giordano Savarin murdered both his mother and father after he had been released from the asylum in Trieste where Basaglia was the director. Basaglia and another colleague were again tried for manslaughter and, again, both were cleared.

Papeschi (1985) presented a more philosophical analysis of Basaglia's writings As Papeschi notes, Basaglia does not seek to deny the existence of mental illness in the way that Szasz (1992) does. Basaglia is fundamentally concerned with the social consequences of the illness for individual patients. Illness leads to forms of 'social violence' being imposed on individuals and the mentally ill as a group. This social violence includes the loss of civil and legal rights and the asylum regime. The asylum regime represents the ultimate manifestation of these forms of social violence. Basaglia, like Foucault is seen as taking a fundamentally nihilist position. Any interventions become forms of management of deviance without any therapeutic aims or outcomes.

It is now over 40 years since the introduction of Law 180. Basaglia died in 1980 at the age of 56, so did not live to see its implementation. Altamura and Goodwin (2010) argue that the introduction of Law 180 has also fundamentally altered the role of the psychiatrist. The closure of public mental health hospitals, it is argued, has reduced the broad scope of 'psychiatry in the community'. Patients with depression and anxiety disorders are now more likely to consult private clinics or psychologists. In addition, Altamura and Goodwin (2010) feel that psychiatrists have lost a range of diagnostic and other skills. They suggest that psychiatrists are involved in the assessment and care of a very limited group of mental disorders – psychotic and related disorders. Professionally, psychiatrists have almost lost their medical identity and become instead bureaucrats.

Foot (2015) notes one of Basaglia's greatest achievement was to reassert the fundamental human dignity of the patients at Gorizia and Trieste. A relational approach was to be the key to revolutionising the regime. Foot (2015: 238) concludes his analysis as follows:

> The basis of his work lay in existentialist philosophy – in particular the work of Jean-Paul Sartre. He believed in trying to understand mentally ill patients by building up a relationship with them, and by 'putting into brackets' the diagnosis that prevents a proper relationship being formed.

Deinstitutionalisation in the US

There are many similarities between the drivers of deinstitutionalisation in the US and the UK. We have seen the importance of key critics of the asylum regime. Goffman (2014) carried out his research in one of the biggest state asylums in the US. This recognition of the abusive nature of the state hospital regime was combined with a recognition that it is better to treat the mentally ill nearer to their families, jobs and communities. In addition, the 1950 and 1960s saw the introduction of new medications that were having an effect on the most severe symptoms. A series of legal decisions restricted the circumstances in which a patient could be admitted on a compulsory basis. Finally, changes in funding under Medicaid, Medicare and Supplemental Security Income allowed states to shift the fiscal burden of the mentally ill to federal agencies. The US has led the way in the expansion of the penal state. It now has roughly 5 per cent of the world's population but over 20 per cent of the world's prison population. There are two important areas to consider. The first is the way that people with mental health problems are drawn into the CJS. The second is the impact of imprisonment on individuals. These are issues that are not unique to the US, but they are perhaps most stark there particularly in some states, the most notable being California. In this section, I will examine the links between the US CJS and mental health systems. I will then go on to discuss the landmark judgement in the case of *Brown v. Plata*. In that case, prisoners in a class action successfully sued the state of California arguing that the overcrowding and poor conditions in prison, including the treatment of the mentally ill, amounted to a breach of their constitutional rights.

In 1963, John F. Kennedy introduced the Community Mental Health Centers Act (Harcourt, 2005; 2011). This legislation envisaged the closure of the federal asylums. As with deinstitutionalisation across the world, the policy was driven by a mixture of progressive idealism and fiscal pragmatism. The conditions in asylums were exposed by journalists and most famously by Wiseman in his 1967 film *Titicut Follies*. Harcourt (2005) notes that while the US prison population remained fairly stable until the advent of the penal state in the 1970s, the number of people institutionalised in psychiatric settings rose from 41,000 to 500,000 in the period 1880–1950. This is a 13-fold increase in a period when the general population rose by a third. Torrey (1997) argued that the increase in the institutionalised population was due to a range of factors including the ageing of the general population, longer stays in hospital and an increased confidence in the role of psychiatry. Additionally, Torrey (1997) suggests that the wider society became less tolerant of deviant behaviour. When he made his announcement, President Kennedy indicated that the institutionalised population would be reduced by a half. The inpatient population was reduced by nearly 60 per cent in the period 1965–75 (Harcourt, 2005). As well as reductions in the overall population, individual asylums became smaller. In 1955 the average mental health institution accommodated 2,000 patients; by 2000, this was down to 500 (Harcourt, 2005, 2011).

The deinstitutionalisation process in the US contained within it a broad shift in attitudes to mental illness. These led to changes in the nature of the psychiatric population. Metzl (2010) demonstrates that this involved a restructuring of the diagnosis of schizophrenia. He argues that having been previously a diagnosis associated with middle and lower middle class white women – symbolised by Virginia Cunningham (Olivia de Havilland) in the 1948 film *The Snake Pit* – it became a diagnosis applied to urban working class black men. Metzl (2010) includes an advert for Haldol in his analysis of the shift in the nature of the diagnosis. The advert has a caricatured figure of a young black man – angry and full of rage, his fists are clenched tight. The headline for the picture is assaultive and belligerent. Harcourt (2005, 2011) concluded that the huge drop in numbers in psychiatric institutions involved a focus on dangerousness and risk. In this context, race became a proxy for risk leading to a sharp increase in the black representation in asylums. Race as a proxy for risk has a long history in the US (Harcourt, 2014) It was further entrenched in the period that saw the expansion of the penal state (Wacquant, 2005; Alexander, 2012). Parsons (2018) demonstrates that deinstitutionalisation is a complex and often highly localised process.

One of the leading most vocal and public critics of deinstitutionalisation in the US has been the psychiatrist and researcher, Professor E. Fuller Torrey. Torrey (1988, 1998, 2010) has long argued that the policy of deinstitutionalisation has been an expensive and catastrophic failure. He argues that the policy has led to the abandonment of the mentally ill. He is particularly critical of the legal decisions that meant the powers to treatment patients against their will were significantly reduced. Torrey has long been an advocate of assertive outpatient treatment (AOT) laws – the US equivalent of community treatment orders (CTOs). An example of this sort of legislation, Kendra's Law – which applies in New York – is discussed in the next section. Torrey has been a keen supporter of groups and campaigns aimed at reversing what he sees as the failures of liberal mental health policies. Torrey is a controversial figure not unlike Szasz but arguing from a very different perspective. Torrey's opponents see him as seeking to undo any progress that has been made in recognising patients' rights. He argues that the pendulum has swung so far as to amount to neglect. The notion here is that the current state of mental health services means that any patients' rights are essentially meaningless.

The CJS has increasingly a site for the provision of mental healthcare (Cummins, 2016). At all stages of the CJS, the mental health status of an individual is a potential factor to consider in the decision-making process. This is the case from an initial beat encounter to sentencing decisions in the Courts. If a person becomes unwell in prison, then the MHA allows for their transfer to forensic mental health services. In outlining his hypothesis, Penrose saw the relationship between the mental health services and CJS as an essentially fluid one – often called 'balloon theory'. Raphael (2000) examined this in the context of the American experience of deinstitutionalisation and the expansion of the penal state. These did not occur in the same time period. The major drop in asylum numbers was completed by 1980 (Harcourt, 2005,

2011) just as the incarceration boom was about to take off. Torrey (2010) found that in 2004–5 there were more than three times more seriously mentally ill persons in jails and prisons than in hospitals. This study (Torrey, 2010) also highlighted significant variations between the states. In North Dakota, there appeared to be roughly equally numbers of mentally ill individuals in prison as hospital. I think that most commentators would agree with Seddon (2009) that it would be impossible to have a situation in which a state could guarantee that there were no mentally ill people in prisons. The aim would be that these numbers are as low as possible and that the most severely mentally ill are transferred to psychiatric facilities at the earliest opportunity. Arizona and Nevada have almost ten times more mentally ill persons in jails and prisons than in hospitals.

Torrey et al (2010) went on to point out that studies suggested that around 16 per cent of inmates in jails and prisons have a serious mental illness. In 1983, the figure was 6.4 per cent. This is a tripling of the figure in a 30-year period. In 1955 there was one psychiatric bed for every 300 Americans. In 2005 there was one psychiatric bed for every 3,000 Americans. It is worth repeating that the prison environment is a totally inappropriate one for someone experiencing severe mental illness. Apart from the fact that it is clearly not a therapeutic environment, there is a great deal of evidence that mentally ill prisoners are more likely to be bullied, assaulted and subject to prison discipline including periods in solitary confinement. Torrey et al (2010) notes that the 1840s reform movement for more humane treatment of the mentally ill, led by Dorothea Dix, was sparked by the appalling conditions in prisons. He argues that events have now come full circle. Deinstitutionalisation has meant the US has now returned to the conditions of the 1840s by putting large numbers of mentally ill people back into jails and prisons.

Raphael and Stoll (2013) noted that in 1996, according to Department of Justice figures, there were 288,000 mentally ill prisoners. At that time, there were 62,000 people in state and county mental hospitals. The over representation of people with mental health problems in CJS continues. The three biggest 'psychiatric facilities' in the US are actually in prisons: Rikers in New York, the Cook County jail and the Los Angeles County Jail system. Raphael and Stoll's (2013) statistical analysis concluded that between 1980 and 2000, the number of people incarcerated as a result of deinstitutionalisation grew from 4.5 to 14 per cent of the general prison population. This study suggested between 28 per cent and 86 per cent of those incarcerated who were suffering from mental illness were in prison because of the failures to establish the community mental health system envisaged in President Kennedy's 1963 speech. They conclude that:

> The findings of this study strongly suggest that the reduction in service capacity of state and county mental hospitals over the past three decades is directly responsible for a large number of mentally ill individuals incarcerated in state prisons. (Raphael and Stoll, 2013: 188)

The US, in many senses, led the charge into the crisis of mass incarceration and its impact on the treatment of the mentally ill. It is also possible that it will lead the way out. Simon (2014) compares mass incarceration to a Biblical flood. The flood is now receding, leaving behind the revelation of the damage that it has done to society, particularly poor urban African American and Hispanic communities. He noted that in *Spain v. Procunier*, the role of prisons was described as to keep 'dangerous men in safe custody under humane conditions'. The reality is somewhat different. Prisoners are more likely to be older or middle aged with associated health problems. The mental and physical health of prisoners is generally much worse than that of the wider society. This is exacerbated by the prison environment. One element of the developing reform movement in the US is fiscal conservatives concerned about the costs of mass incarceration. These costs must meet the increasingly complex healthcare needs of an ageing prison population, including spends on mental health care. There are echoes of deinstitutionalisation, where fiscal conservatives also had a key role.

Notions of rehabilitation disappear in overcrowded jails marked by a daily threat of physical and sexual violence. The brutality which is a central feature of prison life is most apparent in the super-max prison regime. Super-max prisoners such as those at California's massive Pelican Bay Security Housing Unit (SHU) are almost always referred to by authorities as the 'worst of the worst'. These prisoners usually spend 23 hours a day in their cells leaving only for an hour of exercise or showering. Simon (2014) discusses the significance of the case of *Madrid v. Gomez* brought by Pelican Bay SHU prisoners. Judge Thelton's opinion in the case outlines the extreme mental deterioration that solitary confinement eventually produces. It is worth quoting, as Simon does (2014: 50), Judge Thelton's conclusion:

> The overall effect of the SHU is one of stark sterility and unremitting monotony. Inmates can spend years without

ever seeing any aspect of the world except for a small patch of sky. One inmate fairly described the SHU as being 'like a space capsule where one is shot into space and left in isolation'.

In *Brown v. Plata* prisoners sued the state of California. Lawyers for the prisoners successfully argued that the state's penal policies led to the overcrowding in prisons which meant that inadequate health care was provided. Justice Kennedy was so appalled by the conditions that he included photographs in the Supreme Court Judgement. These included examples of overcrowding but also the use of 'dry cells' essentially cages used as holding cells for people waiting for mental health treatment. As Simon (2014: 15) emphasises, Justice Kennedy's opinion also offered some of the strongest language in decades about prisoners as more than legal subjects. They should be treated as possessors of 'human dignity'.

Assertive outpatient treatment and Kendra's Law

One of the key responses to the failings of community care has been the introduction of some form of CTO. These exist now exist in England and Wales, Scotland, New Zealand, Australia, Canada, Israel and in 46 of the United States. There are a variety of models. In England and Wales, patients can only be made subject to a CTO following a long-term compulsory admission. By contrast, in New Zealand, the criteria for an application for a CTO are the same as for a hospital admission. There is an additional requirement that there are appropriate services available and that the social circumstances of the patient mean that a community-based approach is suitable. In New Zealand, the CTO is thus regarded as an alternative to admission while in the England and Wales it is a mechanism to prevent future admissions. The rate of use of CTOs in New Zealand is high by comparison to international use and it is rising. In 2005, the rate was 58 per 100,000 of the general population; by 2011, it was 84 per 100,000 (O'Brien, 2014).

The fundamental arguments in favour of CTOs are that they improve the quality of life of individuals – and by so doing they have a wider positive impact on families and communities. Hospital readmissions would be one measure of their success. Others would include more regular outpatient contact, fewer periods in hospital and reduced contact with the police or other emergency and crisis services (O'Brien, 2014). However, there is a dispute about the claims that this is due to the use of legal coercion. Critics of CTOs argue that these improved outcomes are the result of services meeting their duties and responsibilities. The fact that someone is subject to a CTO means that they are given priority within services. The imposition of the CTO thus has as greater impact on the behaviour of agencies than on those subject to them. The argument against them is that the alleged improved care and support that CTOs produce do not require the restriction of liberty and increased stigma that they entail. In Torrey's memorable phrase, deinstitutionalisation and the failure to provide adequate community mental health services had left people with severe mental health problems 'rotting with their rights on'. The restrictions of assertive outpatient treatment would ensure, it was argued by Torrey, the management of symptoms and better quality of life.

Policy development is driven by a mixture of ideological perspectives, fiscal drivers and also the need to respond to wider political and public concerns. There are many examples of this in the mental health field. Public scandals of various sorts have had a key role in the development of modern mental health policy. Kendra's Law is an example of such a development. In the late 1990s in New York, the media had highlighted a series of incidents of violent crime involving people with mental health problems. On 3 January 1999, Andrew Goldstein, 29, who experienced psychotic illness, murdered Kendra Webdale. Webdale was a 32-year-old aspiring writer, who had come to New York from Buffalo. Goldstein pushed her to her death under a subway train. Goldstein had been admitted to hospital on several occasions. This is awful event came to be seen as emblematic of the failures of deinstitutionalisation. It is also representative of one of the strongest fears in modern urban life: the random attack. Goldstein had been admitted to hospital on several occasions and then discharged without adequate support. The last admission was six weeks before the murder of Kendra Webdale.

Following Goldstein's conviction and sentence to 23 years in prison for second degree murder, there was a campaign for a change in the commitment laws. Eventually, this led to the introduction of Section 9.60 of New York State Mental Health Law – the so-called Kendra's Law. Under its provisions, the court may order assertive outpatient treatment if it finds that:

- the patient is over 18 years of age;
- the patient is suffering from a mental illness;
- the patient is unlikely to survive safely in the community without supervision;

- the patient has a history of lack of compliance with treatment for mental illness.

It is an additional requirement that non-compliance has been a factor in two admissions to hospital within the previous three years or threats of, or actual, violent behaviour or physical harm to self or others within the previous four years.

There are echoes of the Clunis care here (Cummins, 2012). Goldstein had a history of admissions and being discharged without adequate support. An article published in the *New York Times* in May 1999 (Winerup, 1999) showed that Goldstein had been admitted to hospital on 13 occasions. Each admission was voluntary. He was started on medication and each time, when discharged, he moved to live alone in a squalid basement apartment. One of the reasons that social workers and others struggled to find appropriate supported accommodation was long waiting lists, lengthened by severe budget cuts under Governor George Pataki. When Kendra's Law was passed, Pataki earmarked an extra $125 million for the care of the mentally ill.

Kendra's Law was unusual in that it brought with it increased funding (Applebaum, 2005). This funding was to pay for the increased costs of developing more intensive models of case management and to pay for the care of patients who were admitted to hospital. In addition, the law contained a sunset clause which required the reauthorisation of the programme in 2005. It is not surprising that Kendra's Law was subject to a number of legal challenges. The most important of these was the case of K.L. This case was decided by New York's highest court. K.L. had been diagnosed with schizoaffective disorder. He had a history of non-compliance, and violent and aggressive behaviour to his family when he was experiencing psychotic symptoms. K.L., in challenging an AOT order, argued not that he did not meet the criteria rather that the statute was unconstitutional (Applebaum, 2005). The court held that the statute was constitutional only because it lacked any direct mechanisms to enforce compliance with treatment. This is, of course, a pragmatic response to such legislation. Their coercive powers are, in fact, very limited in most cases.

Applebaum (2005) notes that in a five-year period more than 10,000 patients were assessed for their eligibility. There were 4,041 applications for AOTs. These were granted in 93 per cent of cases. The orders are subject to renewal after six months and this occurred in two thirds of cases. The average length of an order was 16 months. The demographic of this group showed that they tended to be single men in their thirties – the mean age was 38. In terms of diagnosis, psychotic disorder was the most common, often complicated by substance use problems. Over the three years before commitment, 97 per cent of patients had been hospitalised, 30 per cent arrested, 23 per cent incarcerated and 19 per cent homeless. The AOT was linked to positive outcomes: arrest, incarceration, psychiatric hospitalisation and homelessness all dropped by between 74 per cent and 87 per cent. Applebaum (2005) that there was a danger of jumping to conclusions about the efficacy of Kendra's Law and AOTs more widely based on this relatively limited study. There are major questions to consider, for example, the sustainability of these improvements when patients are no longer subject to the programme and receiving the support that goes with it.

A mental health scandal in South Africa

In this final section, I will outline the Life Esidimeni scandal in Gauteng Province, South Africa. After the election of the first democratic government and Nelson Mandela as President in 1994, the African National Congress (ANC) was committed to a series of social and welfare reforms to forge a new more equal society and tackle the legacy of colonialism and white rule. The Reconstruction and Development Programme and the Constitution are infused with a rights-based approach and guarantees to protect individual liberty. These moves included a new rights-based approach to health care (Ornellas, 2014). The Mental Health Care Act (Republic of South Africa, 2004) was introduced alongside a National Mental Health Policy Framework and Strategic Plan 2013–2020 (Republic of South Africa, 2009). These new policies were informed by and met international standards on human rights (WHO, 2005). The overarching aim was for the closure of mental hospitals and the establishment of comprehensive community-based mental health services.

The Life Esidimeni scandal is an example of the disastrous implementation of a policy deinstitutionalisation, which led to the deaths of patients. Gauteng is the most populous province of South Africa. It includes Johannesburg and Pretoria. In October 2015, the Department of Health announced that it was terminating its contract with the Life Esidimeni Care Centres, which, at that point, had an estimated 2,000 residents. The termination of the contract meant that the residents would be moved to live in projects run by non-governmental organisations (NGOs), with their families or in psychiatric hospitals. The decision to terminate the contract must be placed in the wider context of South Africa's post-apartheid social policies (Ornellas and Engelbrecht, 2018). These are designed to tackle the legacy of the apartheid regime while promoting a localised rights-based approach. These commitments include a commitment to deinstitutionalisation in mental health care (Makgoba, 2016). It is interesting to note that deinstitutionalisation has, despite its failings, became the standard for progressive mental health policies.

The policy of deinstitutionalisation had been adopted in South Africa from the late 1990s onwards (Ornellas and Engelbrecht, 2018). Deinstitutionalisation has become adopted in over 150 countries across the world so it is not surprising that it was followed in South Africa. In addition, it is seen as a symbol of modernisation and a rights-based approach. Therefore, it has an appeal to emerging democracies. The ending of the Life Esidimeni contract was part of a much broader and deeply embedded policy of deinstitutionalisation (Mngadi, 2017). There was some professional opposition to the moves at the time (Makgoba, 2016). However, on the whole, the policy was seen as a positive move.

The scale of the Life Esidiemeni tragedy was revealed in a report by the Health Ombudsman (Makgoba, 2016). Between October 2015 and June 2016, 1,711 people were 'relocated' from facilities run by Life Esidimeni. The inquiry documented that 144 of these people died – yes, died. The state could not account for the whereabouts of 44 patients; 1,418 who were living in NGO facilities had been subject to the most appalling treatment, which the report concluded amounted to torture. This included being tied up and moved in the back of trucks. The residents had no notice of these moves or where they might be going. They did not have identification documents, which is an important issue given the history of South Africa. Families were not informed of these moves. The Life Esidimeni residents were moved to appalling, often insanitary conditions, and subject to degrading treatment. The Health Ombudsman's report (Makgoba, 2016) estimated that 108 of those who died did so from starvation or dehydration. All 27 NGOs were found to be operating without a licence.

The Ombudsman's report is scathing. It outlines that the NGO facilities were overcrowded. Hygiene was poor; there was low quality or limited food available. These facilities were poorly staffed. There was a lack of qualified mental health staff as well as a lack of access to medicine and other supplies. These facilities admitted more patients than they were allowed. The causes of death were all preventable. Fiscal concerns had definitely been a factor in the decision to terminate the contract. The Ombudsman's report emphasised that this was not acceptable reasoning because it failed to respect the fundamental rights of the patients. The Gauteng Department of Health had failed to develop a plan that would ensure that any savings generated by the termination of the contract would be used for the benefit of patients. This is a finding that can be probably be applied across the majority of deinstitutionalisation schemes that appear in this volume.

The report is clear that the decision to move residents from Life Esidimeni centres was completed in a chaotic fashion. The speed of the changes was a factor in its failure. However, other factors had a role. The residents were simply moved to an environment with limited or no experience of providing community-based mental health services. This lack of infrastructure has been highlighted in the UK and US. Patients were moved from the structured environment of Life Esidimeni into a chaotic one, which was clearly unacceptable. The report concludes that this was not only negligent but also a violation of the human rights of the mentally ill. The Ombudsman concluded that this policy also was also a breach of one of the fundamental principles of health – the preservation of life (Makgoba, 2016).

The scandal that resulted from the closure of the Life Esidimeni might be viewed as such a chaotic and unusual event that there are few, if any, wider conclusions that can be drawn from it. Ornellas and Engelbrecht (2018) disagree strongly with this. They suggest that this is a paradigmatic case of the impact of neoliberal concerns to reduce the size of the social state. In this example, fiscal concerns have led to the most egregious human rights abuse and deaths in appalling circumstances of the poorest and most marginalised. Institutional care was scaled down without any corresponding investment in the community services required to replace it. The progressive language of rights and empowerment masked the fact that the state had simply abandoned individuals.

Conclusion

Policy development is clearly influenced by a number of factors. The historical, political and social contexts all contribute. Given all these factors, one is struck by the similarities between elements of the experiences outlined here. The Gauteng scandal is obviously an outlier in terms of its impact – and the fact that it was exposed so rapidly. However, the causes of the appalling treatment are all present in the experiences of deinstitutionalisation in the US and the UK. These include a hasty and ill-conceived plan for the resettlement of individual patients; and the failure to include service users, their families and carers in these processes. Finally, the state passed on its responsibility for the care of the most vulnerable and marginalised to a poorly regulated and, in this case, negligent independent sector. Alongside structural factors, it is important to acknowledge the role that individuals can play at both a local and national level. Basaglia has remained something of an icon for the anti-psychiatry movement (Foot, 2015; Cummins, 2017). He is an example of the role that charismatic individuals can play in bringing about change but also the potential for it to take place.

8

Neoliberalism, advanced marginality and mental health

Introduction

This chapter will discuss the broader impact of neoliberal social and welfare policy. In particular, it explores the impacts of increased inequality and the spatial concentration of poverty. These processes are referred to as 'advanced marginality'. This concept captures the ways in which areas of poverty are surrounded by areas of affluence. In addition, advanced marginality symbolises the processes whereby groups and individuals are effectively excluded in a literal and metaphorical sense from major areas of modern society. This section is influenced by the work of Loic Wacquant (2008a, 2008b, 2009a, 2009b) and his notion of *territorial stigmatisation*. This is the modern context of community care. It then goes on to examine the impact of austerity policies that have been followed since 2010 on both mental health service users and wider mental health provision. The links between poverty and poor mental health are examined in this section. Increases in inequality have broader impacts in this area. Wilkinson and Pickett (2010, 2018) argue that mental health can be used as one of the measures of inequality. In addition, they argue that polarised societies produce a range of social harms that have negative impacts on individuals and communities. The fundamental argument that I put forward here is that austerity has impacts on individuals' mental health while increasing pressures on statutory and voluntary services. One impact of these processes has been an increase in the use of the MHA, including compulsory admissions to hospital and police involvement in responding to mental health crises. These were among the factors that led to the Wessely Review of the MHA, which was completed in 2018 (Department of Health and Social Care, 2018). There is concern that the wide crisis in mental health services has led to calls for a return to the notion of asylum.

Advanced marginality

Davis (1998) outlined a series of trends in the development of the modern urban environment that served to exclude but also manage poverty and the urban poor. Los Angeles is portrayed by Davis as something of a laboratory for social and economic policies such as the management of public space. His classic work has a prophetic quality. The trends that he identified have intensified and become more widespread over the past 25 years. One result is that poverty has become increasingly spatially (and racially) concentrated. The focus in this work is on the urban environment but these trends can also be observed in rural settings. Wacquant (2009a, 2009b) outlines the way that the contraction of the welfare state under neoliberal influenced governments means that communities are denied access to decent housing, education and employment opportunities. Wacquant (2008a, 2008b, 2009a, 2009b) sees these changes as a key feature of neoliberal social policies. He uses the term advanced marginality as a counter to the New Right term 'underclass', a term possibly most associated with Charles Murray (1990). Murray sees poverty in individual, essentially moral, rather than structural terms (Cummins, 2018). Advanced marginality is an endogenous feature of neoliberalism (Wacquant, 2016). It should be viewed as an inevitable outcome of the attacks on the features of the social state that had been established by post war Keynesian economic and social policies. Alongside these developments, there has been a shift to more punitive approaches to welfare. People with long-term mental health problems because of the barriers they face in the labour market are greatly affected by these changes.

There were clearly several problems with the exclusionary nature of the post war social democratic settlement. It was based on a series of gendered, racial and class assumptions. Neoliberalism produces inequality, social and racial exclusion alongside an expansion in precarious employment (Standing, 2011). The final element of these processes is the expansion in the penal state. The US and the UK have both seen huge expansions in the use of imprisonment (Gottschalk, 2006; Alexander, 2012; Simon, 2014; Cummins, 2017). Prisoners are overwhelmingly young men from poor, marginalised urban backgrounds and neighbourhoods. This fact adds to the stigma that such communities already face (Clear, 2009; Drucker, 2011). The CJS has become increasingly a de facto provider of certain forms of mental health care. The trends outlined here mean that people with mental health problems are increasingly drawn into the CJS.

The nature of the welfare state

Garland (2014) notes that it is generally opponents of the welfare state who use the term pejoratively. All states are welfare states in the sense that they play some role in the provision of welfare and essential services to citizens. In addition, all welfare systems include disciplinary aspects. The neoliberal retooling of the state in the US and the UK has seen a significant move towards more punitive approaches in several fields. Conditionality has been a feature of all modern welfare states. The 1834 Poor Law Amendment Act enshrined the principle of less eligibility in law. This meant that conditions in the workhouse had to be harsh with the specific aim of deterring those who might wish to claim relief. The welfare reforms which I will go on to outline are a modern manifestation of a recurring set of opinions – the poor are lazy and indolent, have too many children and are keen to sponge of the state. Variants of these attitudes can be found in popular, academic and policy discourse across the ages (Welshman, 2013).

Bourdieu (1998) outlined what he termed the Right and Left Hands of the state. On the Right Hand were agencies concerned with social order – the police, courts and prisons. On the Left Hand were what we might term welfare agencies. There are some difficulties with this reductionist analysis (Garrett, 2007). A polar presentation of the role of state agencies ignores a more complex reality. This is clearly apparent in the mental health sphere. I am sure that my social work colleagues and students would place social work on the Left Hand. However, social workers are part of systems that involve the exercise of legal powers to intervene in the lives of citizens against their will – for example in the fields of child protection and mental health. In the same way, agencies such as the police, which Bourdieu places on the Right Hand of the state, also play a welfare role. For example, mental health work is increasingly an important part, possibly as much as 20 per cent, of police work in the UK (Centre for Mental Health, 2008). It is, thus, increasingly difficult to categorise the role of several state agents in a binary fashion – welfare versus punitive or disciplinary interventions. It should be noted here that there is another approach in the mental health field that would suggest that all the interventions, whatever they are termed – welfare, therapeutic, medical or social work – are fundamentally exercises in power and social control.

The complexities of these welfare and other policies are played out in the interactions between individual citizens and the state employees in offices and houses across the country daily. Lipsky (2010) acknowledges that this means that public workers are thus in a position where they can subvert or resist policies (Barnes and Prior, 2009.) Bourdieu et al (1999: 184) see this as a form of collective double consciousness. Social work is thus 'shot through with the contradictions of the State'. Its professional value base commits social workers to a set of progressive values based on notions of human dignity and social justice. At the same time, many individuals and families experience social work interventions as harsh and punitive or as overriding their rights and wishes. These tensions are played out at both the individual and organisational levels.

Austerity

Since the early 1990s, the right has mounted a protracted 'war of position' against the key features of a universalist welfare state (Garrett, 2017). One key element of this is the way that the term welfare has come to have overwhelmingly negative connotations. Wacquant (2009a) traces the nexus between academics, right-wing think-tanks and opinion pieces in Conservative-supporting newspapers that have helped to shift the meaning and usage of the term. Slater's (2018) analysis of the development and use of the term 'sink estate' is a case study analysis of these processes. In contrast to the 'national emergency' discourse of the coalition, it is possible to see austerity as a class project that seeks to recast the UK welfare state. This recasting would remove any last vestiges of Scandinavian social democratic welfare approaches, leaving US style residual forms of provision. The UK leaving the EU will weaken the social protections of workers further. However, there is an alternative which sees these processes as more fragmented involving continual struggles across political, economic, symbolic and social spaces (Wacquant, 2013).

Austerity politics has seen a hardening of social attitudes. Sayer (2015) notes that the financial crash, while leading to some limited social criticisms of bankers, has also paradoxically led a hardening of anti-welfarism. This is the result of the way that the coalition government was able to construct and successfully maintain a narrative that the crisis in the public finances was the result of welfare spending. There is an important proviso here in that welfare was very much referring to benefits paid to those who were out of work rather than pensions. Jensen and Tyler (2015: 471) argue that the result has been the development of a new form of political economy which involves what they term a 'hardening of anti-welfare commonsense'.

It is now over ten years since the banking crisis of 2008. The initial response to that crisis was for government to spend huge sums of public money to bail out financial institutions. The banks were 'too big to fail'. In the UK, the Brown administration followed standard Keynesian economics by attempting to stimulate demand in the economy. These measures included a reduction in VAT and increased capital spending. These policies came to an end with the formation of the coalition government in 2010. Coalition governments are very rare in UK modern political history. The coalition presented itself as a government formed in response to a national emergency. The emergency was the position of the government finances, but the cause of that position was presented as the previous Labour government's profligacy. In introducing a series of cuts to public spending and social welfare programmes, the Conservative Chancellor of Exchequer, George Osborne, claimed that 'we are all in this together' (*Guardian*, 2012). Brown (2015) noted that calls to individual sacrifice are an integral part of the discourse of the fiscal crisis as national emergency. Reductions in welfare spending inevitably have the greatest impact on the poorest and most vulnerable members of society. These are the groups that are most reliant on public services. The scale of the cuts in welfare spending represent a huge retrenchment in and recasting of the welfare state. Beatty and Fothergill (2016) calculated that welfare spending will be reduced by £27 billion a year by 2020–21. The work of Emejulu and Bassel (2015) demonstrates that austerity's impacts are racialised and gendered. Crossley (2016) concluded that the largest cuts were experienced in those areas that had officially been identified as being poorer and having increased local needs.

Austerity was presented as its supporters as a technocrat exercise in macroeconomic management. This cloaks the fundamental retooling of the welfare state that it entailed (Goodman, 2018). Austerity policies had resulted in the UK public sector becoming the smallest among major economies (Taylor-Gooby, 2012). This includes the US. This period of retrenchment is the most sustained cutting of social provision that the modern welfare state has faced (Taylor-Gooby, 2012). It went beyond what the Thatcher governments of the 1980s had thought politically possible (Young, 2013). Neoliberal opposition to the welfare state has consistently presented it as profligate and creating dependency (Cummins, 2018). The allegedly generous nature of UK welfare provision was, in this analysis, the cause of the UK's fiscal difficulties in 2010 – not the bailing out of the banks. In fashioning what the prime minister termed a 'smarter state' (Cameron, 2015), austerity involved the attempted recasting of the relationship between individuals, communities and the state.

In November 2018, Professor Philip Alston, United Nations Special Rapporteur on extreme poverty and human rights visited the UK and wrote a devastating report on the impact of austerity policies. The report (Alston, 2018) demonstrates the way that austerity policies have shredded the social welfare safety net. The report notes that the UK is the fifth largest economy in the world. However, as a result of austerity, 14 million people – one fifth of the population – are living in poverty. The impact of the development and life chances of children and young people is described as 'not just a disgrace but a social calamity and an economic disaster, all rolled into one'. The Alston report argues that austerity has seen the ripping up of the post war Beveridge social contract. Todd (2015) notes that the previous period of austerity in the UK, which followed the Second World War, saw the establishment of key features of the modern welfare state such as the National Health Service (NHS). This period of austerity has seen the fragmentation and marketisation of key welfare institutions such as the NHS and the deprofessionalisation of the staff who work in them.

The UN Rapporteur paints a very bleak picture of the damage that austerity policies have inflicted on local services. This includes, for example, the closure of 500 children's centres in 2010–15; 340 libraries were closed with the loss of 8,000 jobs in 2010–16. These are the sorts of services that have a vital but often hidden role in local communities. Legal aid has been significantly reduced, meaning that access to justice has become even more dependent on having the necessary financial resources. The changes in legal aid have had the overall impact of effectively denying poorer people representation in key areas of public law such as family, housing and immigration (Bowcott and Duncan, 2018). Such services are of even greater importance to poorer families and communities. The UN report suggests that the overall impact of such changes will result in the loss of the protections of the European Charter of Fundamental Rights.

Austerity policies in the UK have continued an existing trend of increased conditionality within the welfare system. Austerity has been combined with the introduction of Universal Credit (UC). UC is presented as a way of simplifying the notorious complex system of benefits so that there is one payment. However, the introduction of the system has been marked by logistical difficulties. The UN Rapporteur's report highlights the way that UC is the first service that is 'digital by default' – the whole system is online. This wrongly assumes that all claimants are digitally literate and have access to the internet. The libraries that remain open have seen a huge upsurge in customers needing support with dealing with UC online. For example, according to the UN Rapporteur's report, in Newcastle staff aided nearly 2000 customers in a year around these issues. The other important aspect of UC is the delay in payment. UC is paid monthly in arrears. This means that a claimant has to wait one calendar month from the date they submitted their application before their first UC payment is made. There is then a delay in the payment to reaching the claimant's bank account. It can take up to five weeks before the first payment is received. This means that many claimants are in arrears or facing financial hardship from day one. This is not an accidental outcome; it is built into the UC system.

Alongside these developments, austerity has strengthened the trends towards a more punitive approach to welfare. New rules meant that those claiming benefits were subject to sanctions – reductions in or cessation of payments imposed on claimants who do not meet conditions such as attending job centre meetings. The Work Capability Assessment (WCA) scheme meant that individuals who were claiming the Employment and Support Allowance (ESA) underwent a fitness to work assessments. Barr et al (2015) concluded that the WCA process was linked to: 590 suicides; 279,000 additional cases of self-reported mental health problems; and 725,000 additional prescriptions for anti-depressants. The WCA regime applies to people with physical health problems. Ryan (2015) reported on 80 cases where people died having been found 'fit for work'.

Austerity's architects may have presented it as a response to a national emergency. However, its main aim of shrinking the role of the welfare state places it firmly in the libertarian tradition that flows from Hayek (2014) and Friedman (2009). The demonisation of the poor as feckless and work-shy shares key elements with Murray (1990). In fact, its roots can be traced back to Booth's (1890) representation of poverty in Victorian London (Cummins, 2018). Welshman (2013) demonstrates the way that so-called problem families and communities have been rediscovered and redefined at regular intervals ever since. In this tradition, poverty is regarded not as a structural issue. Its causes are the individual moral failings of the poor. Clarke and Newman (2012) term the way that the fundamentally structural issues of poverty and economic inequality are transformed into a discourse of welfare dependency and the burden on the state as the 'alchemy of austerity'. Mills (2018) in her analysis of the reporting of suicides linked to austerity and benefit reforms demonstrates the way that these cases are presented as individual tragedies. They are depoliticised. The broader context of the government policy that lie behind these cases is ignored or downplayed. Grover (2018) sees austerity as a manifestation of what Engels termed social murder. Social murder encapsulates the way that the lives of working class were shortened by the consequences of economic and social inequalities that are the inevitable consequence of social relations of capitalism. Cooper and Whyte (2017) describe austerity as a form of 'institutional violence' — it is carried out in a bureaucratic form. This is not to minimise the damage that it does, rather it emphasises that it occurs on a daily basis out of sight. Cooper and Whyte (2017) also emphasised the brutal, violent nature of the impact of austerity, and that this represents 'slow violence'. Potentially, the most damaging effects of austerity will be felt in the medium or long term. Austerity should be placed firmly in wider developments of later modern capitalism that has led to increases in social and economic inequality. Bauman, in an interview with the *Guardian*, noted that we underestimate the pain of humiliation, being denied the value of your worth and identity and of how you earned your living and kept your commitments to your family and neighbours (Bunting, 2003).

The conclusion of the UN Rapporteur's report is emphatic. Austerity was a clear political choice. In addition, the poorest and most vulnerable individuals and communities will bear the brunt of the impact of these policies. The shift in welfare reforms have led to a situation where 'British compassion for those are suffering has been replaced by a punitive, mean spirited and callous approach apparently designed to instill discipline…' (Alston, 2018: 3).

It is a fairly obvious point but one worth repeating: these policies have the most impact on those living in poverty. People with health problems, including mental problems, are overrepresented in this group. Another obvious point worthy of repetition is that people living in poverty have fewer resources to respond to personal and family crises. Both these points seem to have been ignored by the architects of austerity and welfare reform. At the same time, welfare and community services are under increasing financial pressures having to respond to increased demand within a context of reduced budgets.

One of the most significant shifts in recent years has been the recognition that social and life experiences have a role in the development of mental health problems. In addition, the impact of mental health diagnosis, illness and stigma can have an impact on the economic and other opportunities that people with mental health problems can face. There is a social gradient in the extent of mental health problems – the impact of severe mental illness means that many individuals are unable to work or, if they can return to work, they find it difficult to gain employment because of discrimination. Macintyre et al (2018) argued that there should be a closer focus on the links between social economic factors and mental health problems. Such a move would be a two-pronged approach looking at both causal factors but also social implications. Shim et al (2014) suggest that though there have been moves in this direction, medical and individualised approaches to mental distress continued to dominate. Macintyre et al (2018), echoing the approach of Basaglia, concluded a social justice approach in the mental health field has to start with a socioeconomic analysis.

Very few commentators would now take a 'purely medical model' approach to the causes, onset and impact of mental illness. For example, Sir Robin Murray, a leading British psychiatrist perhaps best known for his work on the links between cannabis use and schizophrenia, was asked about mistakes he had made in his long and distinguished career. His reply was that it was to underestimate social, economic, political and cultural factors when examining mental health outcomes (Murray, 2017). The links between poverty, inequality and poor mental health are clear. However, there is much debate about the way that potential causal factors and poor mental health outcomes play out (Marmot, 2010). Living in poverty should be viewed as a stressful experience (Cummins, 2018). It is broadly acknowledged that acute stress has a negative impact on individual mental health (Wilkinson and Pickett, 2017). As well as these impacts, it is important to acknowledge that there remains a huge stigma attached to mental illness. This is despite more open social attitudes in this area and public awareness raising campaigns. Stigma remains a key factor in the development of health inequalities (Hatzenbuehler et al, 2013).

The moves towards community care were, in part, based on an idealised view of community life. In this model, communities are supportive environments. Whether this was ever the case is open to doubt. However, it is clear that neoliberal social and welfare policies followed by a period of austerity have placed tremendous pressures on communities. The World Health Organisation (WHO) (2014) in outlining the social determinants of mental health makes it clear that economic factors have to be considered alongside social, political, cultural and historical ones. This approach requires a focus on both individuals and the communities in which they are living. For example, Rehman (2016) in examining the rates of suicide in Maskwacis, a reserve of the Cree Nation in Canada, looks at not only current issues such as poverty, unemployment and substance misuse but also Canada's colonial history. These factors combine to produce the mental health crisis the community faces (Rehman, 2016).

There is a range of socioeconomic factors, such as income inequality, poor housing and living in communities with a lack of resources, that impact on mental health (Silva et al, 2016). Lower socioeconomic status has been linked with suicidal behaviour (Platt et al, 2017). There are other forms of marginalisation that have an impact on mental health. For example, asylum seekers and refugees or those who have experienced other forms of trauma, are more vulnerable to the development of mental health problems (Rafferty et al, 2015). Topor and Ljungqvist's (2017) research with service users demonstrates the positive impact of relatively small increases income can have. The increased income 'impacted their sense of self through experiences of mastery, agency, reciprocity, recognition and security'. Eaton's (1980) 'social drift' hypothesis suggests that the onset of severe mental illness and its potential social consequences such as loss of employment and hospitalisation led to lower socioeconomic status.

A health inequalities approaches argues that the roots of many of the issues that we now classify as mental illness fundamentally have their roots in poverty, social inequality and injustice (Marmot, 2010; Karban, 2016). The impact of austerity has been to deepen inequalities. Bourdieu et al (1999) concluded that the poorest areas of our cities become characterised by 'absence': they have been largely abandoned by the welfare institutions of the state. Austerity has had a profound impact on the welfare state and those who are most reliant on the services it provides. The coalition government's policies, therefore, inevitably had the most impact on the most vulnerable. Fifty per cent of the cuts in spending fell in two areas: benefits and local government spending (Centre for Welfare Reform, 2015).

One of the major planks of austerity economics has been the imposition of more conditions on those claiming out of work or disability benefits. It should be noted that the introduction of reforms such as WCA built on those introduced by the Labour government of Gordon Brown. The WCA was introduced in 2008. Originally, the scheme was managed by a private IT company ATOS who won the contract from the Department of Work and Pensions (DWP), the government department responsible for these issues. The WCA is still outsourced to Maximus, a private organisation, which carries out the assessment for the DWP. The WCA scheme was presented by the DWP as an attempt to help people off benefits and into employment. In the assessment process, there are three possible outcomes: fit for work;

unfit for work but fit for pre-employment training; and fit for neither work nor training. The WCA was applied to those claiming benefits on the grounds of physical disabilities but also mental health problems.

The WCA assessment is essentially a purely functional one. This is problematic in all cases but particularly those who experience mental health issues. Mental health problems are complex and fluctuating, meaning that a functional type assessment will not capture the real impact of difficulties on individuals. The WCA assessments are often carried out by staff with little understanding or professional experience of mental health problems. The impact on an individual's ability to work may vary across various forms of employment. It will also change because of the nature of the difficulties that they face. For example, low mood or anxiety are symptoms of illness that would be difficult to evidence in the way that bureaucracies demand. All these factors combine to put people with mental health problems at a disadvantage in this process.

Alongside the potential impact of the WCA process on individuals – people being found fit for work when they were not – the wider impact of the whole process needs to be considered. Barr et al (2015) examined the programme in the period 2010–13. The authors concluded that, across England, the WCA process was linked to: 590 suicides; 279,000 additional cases of self-reported mental health problems; and 725,000 additional prescriptions for anti-depressants Those in the lowest socioeconomic groups are more likely to be in receipt of these benefits. The social gradient in health (Marmot, 2010) means there is a greater prevalence of mental and physical health problems within this cohort. Any reductions in welfare spending are likely to be outweighed by the personal and wider damage that the policy caused. It may have led to increased public spending in terms of greater calls on mental health and other agencies.

Austerity economic policies have not been limited to the UK. Even more extreme policies were imposed on Greece following the Eurozone crisis. The conditions attached to the bailout included significant cuts in welfare and pensions. These cuts had huge impacts on individuals, families and communities. Pensions and other benefits were cut by up to 25 per cent. Prior to the economic crisis, Greece had one of the lowest suicide rates in the EU. In April 2012, Greece was shocked by the suicide of a 77-year-old pensioner, a retired pharmacist who shot himself outside the parliament building in Athens. In a note, he stated that he had decided to end his life as he did not want to be reduced to foraging in bins for food. The suicide encapsulated the despair of many of the older generation in Greece. The shredding of the social state has clear negative impacts on health outcomes (Stuckler and Basu, 2013). Antonakakis and Collins (2016) explored the relationship between austerity and suicide. The paper examines trends across Greece, Italy, Ireland, Portugal and Spain. Fiscal austerity has had an impact on the suicide rate in these countries. The study concluded that these policies of retrenchment have short-, medium- and long-term impacts on the suicide rates of males. A 1 per cent reduction in government spending is associated with increases of 1.38 per cent, 2.42 per cent and 3.32 per cent in the short-, medium- and long-term male suicide rates, respectively.

The Mental Health Act

Despite the changes in mental health legislation, the use of coercive legal powers casts a long shadow over mental health services. There are no other areas of medicine where doctors use legal powers to treat their patients against their will on such a regular basis. The obtaining of informed consent is one of the corner stones of modern medical ethics. Mental health remains an exception. One of the criticisms of the Wessely Review was that it failed to adequately consider this issue. There is an implicit assumption in the progressive arguments for community care that the use of compulsory powers will be significantly reduced if not disappear completely. Despite a strong official rhetoric about greater service user involvement and joint decision making, this has not been the case. As noted earlier, one of the reasons given for the establishment of the Wessely Review was the increased use of powers under the MHA.

The use of compulsory powers under the MHA has been on an upward trend for some time – virtually the whole period covered by this book. There are several factors at play here. The reduction in the number of beds means that the most severely ill cohort of patients will be admitted. It is possible to argue that the rise in the use of the MHA should be viewed as a positive as it at least establishes a system of rights and protections for patients. Against this, one has to balance the negative impact of the experience of being detained. This is an under researched area. More work needs to be done to examine this – I would argue from all perspectives: those of service users, families and carers and mental health professionals. Based on information collected via the NHS Digital online on Omnibus KP90 collection system, in 2015/16 there were 63,662 detentions under the MHA, an increase of 9 per cent from the 2014/15 figure of 58,399. This is quite a staggering statistic. If we take a longer perspective, we can see that the 2015/16 figures represent virtually a 50 per cent rise in detentions from the 2005/06 figure of 43,361 detentions. If these trends continue, the 2025/26 figure would be pushing towards 100,000 uses of the MHA.

On 31 March 2016, 5,954 patients were detained in private hospitals (not relating to admissions under Sections 2 and 3), showing that the private sector has taken on an increasing role in the provision of mental health care. Pressure on the NHS has meant that there has been an increase in the use of beds in private hospitals. This figure of 5,954 represents 30 per cent of all detained patients. This is the highest percentage since 2006, when 17 per cent of patients were detained in private hospitals. There has been a particularly significant increase in the use of Section 3 following an initial admission under Section 2. In 2015/16, there were 12,462 such incidences. This represents an increase of over 80 per cent on the previous four years. There were 4,361 CTOs were issued in 2015/16. This was a decrease of 4 per cent compared with the 4,564 issued in 2014/15. There were 2,294 recalls to hospital, a slight fall compared with 2014/15. In 2015/16, there were 3,120 either revocation or discharges of CTOs (Care Quality Commission, 2018). At the end of March 2016, there were 25,577 people subject to the provisions of the MHA. Of these, 20,151 were detained in hospitals and 5,954 of these were detained in private hospitals. Keown et al (2018) in their analysis of trends in the use of the MHA concluded that paradoxically community care had led to significant rises in the use of compulsory powers. They argued that this was partly the result of better case management and a clearer focus on risk management and partly it was due to changes in legislation. The study also noted that there was an increase in the use of private providers of publicly funded care – a pattern that is familiar from other eras of mental health policy.

Policing and mental health

The role of the police in mental health work has become the focus of increased debate. These have been heightened by the impact of austerity. The number of police officers has fallen while the demands have increased. Within the organisational culture of policing, mental health work can be seen as 'not proper policing'. The image of policing in the media and popular culture is very much dominated by responses to serious crime. This brings with it a sort of glamour somewhat at odds with the day-to-day reality of policing (Cummins et al, 2014). There is a danger that mental health work will be seen as having a lower status and organisational priority. Responding to a mental health emergency or other situations involving a vulnerable adult requires a different and softer set of skills than tackling street crime does. These are complex issues which are not easily resolved. One of the frustrations for officers is that they are often called to the same address on numerous occasions (Cummins and Edmondson, 2016)

Policing has always had a welfare role (Bittner, 1967, 1970). This has increased during the period of deinstitutionalisation. The Bradley Review (2008) and the Home Affairs Select Committee Report (2015) both highlighted concerns about the increasing demands being placed on the police. In October 2018, the House of Commons Home Affairs Committee published *Policing for the Future*. The report is based on evidence taken from a range of witnesses including Chief Constables and Chief Inspector Michael Brown. Dee Collins, Chief Constable of West Yorkshire Police, in giving evidence stated that '83% of my time in terms of delivering services is not about crime'. The report highlights three areas where the demands on the police are increasingly complex and demanding: mental health work, missing people (particularly missing children) and multi-agency child protection work. In situating this work in the wider context of modern policing, the inquiry highlighted that:

> A prominent theme emerging throughout this inquiry was the increasing volume of police work arising from identifying and managing various forms of vulnerability, including safeguarding vulnerable adults who cross their path, being first-on-scene during a mental health crisis, undertaking child protection work on a multi-agency basis, and dealing with repeat missing person incidents, including looked-after children. (House of Commons Home Affairs Select Committee, 2018: 53)

One of the ongoing issues in this field is problems with defining exactly what constitutes mental health work and then collecting relevant data. In his evidence, Chief Inspector Brown told the committee that the data does not lead easily from police systems that were built for purposes such as crime recording. Despite these difficulties in robust data collection, the overall trends are clear. The BBC reported (Greenwood, 2017) that a freedom of information (FOI) request showed that 23 police forces in England and Wales dealt with 215,000 mental health cases in 2016–17 – a 39 per cent increase on the year before. Some forces saw demand in this area doubled.

The use of Section 136

Section 136 MHA is a police power. It authorises any police officer to remove someone who appears to be mentally disordered from a public place to a 'place of safety'. A 'place of safety' is broadly defined but is usually a hospital or a police cell. This is an emergency power and is generally used in circumstances where a person is considered to be putting themselves at immediate risk. The use of Section 136 MHA relies on the assessment of the individual police officers involved. There is no need for a formal medical diagnosis. The purpose of Section 136 is for a mental health assessment to be carried out by a psychiatrist and an Approved Mental Health Professional (AMHP). The place of safety should normally be a hospital-based setting. Most mental health trusts have created specially designated areas – Section 136 suites – where the formal assessments can take place.

The use of Section 136 MHA has become something of a measure of the extent of police involvement in mental health work. As noted, it is a rather crude measure as it ignores very significant areas of police work, for example vulnerable adults in police custody. As the law stands at the moment, the police are the only agency that have the powers to intervene in emergency situations. Having acknowledged that the police have a much broader role in mental health work, the use of Section 136 MHA can be viewed as an indicator of the pressures on both individuals and community services. The rise in its use shows that the police are being called to respond to more individuals experiencing acute mental distress. As with the use of other compulsory powers, the rise in the use of Section 136 MHA is quite startling. In the year to March 2016, there were 22,965 uses of Section 136 MHA in England and Wales (BBC News, 2019). This represented an increase of 18 per cent to in the year to March 2016. There was a fall in the use of police cells as a place of safety from 3,996 individuals to 1,764.

The issues of race and mental health have been prominent in the era of community care. The use of Section 136 MHA is another area that highlights the concerns about the over-representation of BAME groups, particularly young black men (Rogers and Faulkner, 1987; Dunn and Fahy, 1990; Bhui et al, 2003). This is a crucial issue as it means that in a number of cases the first contact that this group has with mental health services is via the police or other areas of the CJS. Section 136 MHA is much more likely to take place outside standard office hours when normal support services are less likely to be available. Borschmann et al (2010) indicate that the 'typical' Section 136 patient is a young, single working class male with a history of mental illness. This is the group in the population that is least likely to access general health care or be registered with a GP. The limited research that examines service user perspectives emphasises that being subject to Section 136 MHA is experienced as a custodial rather than a therapeutic intervention (Jones and Mason, 2002; Riley et al, 2011).

Conclusion

Social work interventions are much more likely to take place in poorer communities. These interventions, despite the best efforts of social workers, are increasingly experienced as punitive rather than supportive. The economic policies of neoliberalism have increasingly concentrated power and resources in the hands of elites. At the same time, the social state has been, to use Giroux's (2011) term, 'shredded'. Karban (2016) shows that the areas of the social state that have been hardest hit are also the ones that have the greatest protective mental health influence. The state has reduced funding to agencies and voluntary sector organisations and other groups that can act as a buffer between it and individuals and families. The development of deinstitutionalisation began as these policies, which have done the greatest damage to community bonds, were being introduced. Government fiscal imperatives and a progressive discourse were present, but it was readily apparent which would have the most influence on policy development.

Neoliberalism is a political, economic and class project that has at its core a view that the 'market' and the alleged disciplines of the market have to be applied across as many areas of society as possible. This flooding of the market into all areas means that other values such as mutuality, reciprocity and a respect for the individual are pushed to the margins, or struggle to survive in a hostile environment. In the neoliberal schema, markets reward success. In a neatly circular argument, these rewards are always justified because they are determined by the market. Success is always seen in monetary terms and is individual in its nature. In addition, success is based on individual effort, skill or vision or a combination of the three. These core beliefs are at the heart of the neoliberal distrust in the modern welfare state. From this perspective, the state and its bureaucracies are naturally inefficient. This anti-statism is, perhaps, most apparent in attitudes towards the welfare state. It is characterised as monolithic and dependency producing. It rewards or actively encourages anti-social behaviour. The final argument against the welfare state is that it costs too much and that it is paid for by taxation. The burden of that taxation falls on the middle and upper classes who are least likely to use these services. These trends came together under the umbrella of 'austerity'.

The UK has become a more divided and polarised society over the past 30 years. Alongside this increase in inequality, the public discourse has harshened, fuelled by tabloid media attacks on those living in poverty. The work of Tyler (2013), Jensen and Tyler (2015) and others demonstrates the ways in which tabloid media and reality TV programmes have helped shape an anti-welfare, anti-poor discourse. The advent of reality TV and poverty porn has also created an environment which presents those living in poverty and their daily struggles against this marginality as a form of entertainment. The same media outlets that had such a key role in undermining community care in the 1980s and 1990s by fuelling a moral panic about stranger attacks have played a key role in supporting austerity. Austerity has been a series of policies that, as the UN Rapporteur's report (Alston, 2018) makes clear, has done huge social damage.

9

Conclusion

So we beat on, boats against the current, borne back ceaselessly into the past.

F. Scott Fitzgerald, *The Great Gatsby*

This volume has examined the impacts of deinstitutionalisation and community care. These are two aspect of the shift in mental health policy in the past 60 years. I argue that these need to be analysed but are fundamentally connected. The asylum and the community were often presented in a rather limited and concrete fashion as polar opposites of each other. The failings of the asylum regime would disappear in community settings. If there is one lesson from the deinstitutionalisation process it is that all the failings and abuses of the asylum regime have appeared in one modified form or another in community settings. This is most dramatically apparent in the various inquiries and reports that appear in this volume. The Gauteng scandal is the most extreme example of this. However, we witness other examples – such as homeless individuals who are clearly experiencing some form of mental distress – on a daily basis. This raises a more fundamental question about investment in mental health services and the social state more generally.

There are two clear strands to the development of deinstitutionalisation: fiscal conservatism, concerned with the cost of all state welfare provision, including mental health services; and a civil rights approach to the treatment of the mentally ill. By the 1980s, the long-stay mental hospitals were no longer sustainable. This was because of an acceptance that the care they provided was, overall, inadequate. In the UK, the Thatcher government, when it introduced the NHS and Community Care Act (1990), was clear that the economic policies of the government meant that new funding arrangements were demanded. The optimistic view that the abuses of the institutions would be replaced by mental health services founded on civic notions did not survive in the harsh political and economic climate of that period. The government and wider policy responses focused on organisational and audit issues.

In his discussion of Foucault's lectures that were published as *The Birth of the Biopolitics*, Garrett (2018) notes that neoliberalism is now a contested term. For some, it has become a concept that has lost genuine theoretical, conceptually or analytical value. Garrett (2018) notes that critics suggest that neoliberalism is used as an explanation for all of society's ills. This is, of course, a very limited analysis. One obvious criticism being that it assumes that there was a glorious period of social progress before the arrival of the Thatcher and Reagan governments. Dunn (2017) notes that the term has most traction in academia and among 'left elites'. One of the lessons of deinstitutionalisation is that economic factors can be combined with seemingly opposed social values to support changes in welfare policy. There is rarely a sole explanation for the development of social policy. One must examine a range of factors: social, cultural, economic and political, alongside other pressures such as the media reporting of a scandal or abuse. Other writers have continued to find the term useful as an analytical tool. Bourdieu (2001) saw neoliberalism as a 'conservative revolution' that sought to overthrow the post war social democratic consensus, a view shared by politicians such as Thatcher and Reagan with the focus being on the maximisation of profits. This requires the extension of the market to all areas of life and as the monetisation of human activity and relationships (Harvey, 2005; Brown, 2015). Neoliberalism is committed to a small state and personal freedom. The economic and political are intertwined here. Giroux (2011) highlights the way that neoliberal ideas have been able to set the agenda across social, political, economic and cultural fields. Bauman (2007) describes a culture of 'hyperindividualism' which leads to a loosening and weakening of social and community ties. From the 1980s onwards, the role of the state has undergone a radical change. The expansion of the market or market mechanisms into a range of areas has seen the state become an equal player – in the jargon 'a stakeholder' – alongside others. One can thus see the overlaps between a philosophy committed to the reduction of the state and progressive ideas that focus on individualism and choice.

Fraser (2017) in her analysis of the rise of Trump and the Brexit vote argued that these shifts marked the end of what she termed 'progressive neoliberalism'. She used this term as a way to capture the processes whereby neoliberalism had co-opted mainstream currents of new social movements. This can be seen in the way that huge global corporations, such as Apple, Facebook and Amazon, present themselves as dynamic and committed to key issues such as diversity while at the same time engaging in anti-social behaviour such as selling private data and avoiding paying corporate tax. Fraser (2017) suggests that these organisations and governments have used the language of social movements such as feminism and anti-racism – diversity, choice, empowerment. The Blair and Clinton administrations were the leaders in this shift. Fraser (2017) sums it up thus:

> Clinton was the principal engineer and standard-bearer of the 'New Democrats,' the U.S. equivalent of Tony Blair's 'New Labor.' In place of the New Deal coalition of unionized manufacturing workers, African Americans, and the urban middle classes, he forged a new alliance of entrepreneurs, suburbanites, new social movements, and youth, all proclaiming their modern, progressive bona fides by embracing diversity, multiculturalism, and women's rights. Even as it endorsed such progressive notions, the Clinton administration courted Wall Street.

Mental health policy as outlined in this volume can be viewed as an early example of progressive neoliberalism.

The criticisms of community care did not take that long to emerge. Leff (1997) demonstrated that the early resettlement programmes of long-stay patients could be managed successfully. These schemes were, on the whole, better planned and resourced. Leff (1997) highlighted that community-based provision was marginally more expensive than institutionalised care. The progressive argument for community care was never about reducing costs. It was based on a rather naïve assumption that the level of investment in mental health services would remain the same. The funds would be spent on a range of community mental health provision. This period was relatively short lived. One of the key lessons that can be drawn from deinstitutionalisation is the need to build community services at the same time as closing asylums. In the examples that are examined here, there are very few circumstances where this occurred. The result is that community services were and continue to play catch up. There are too many examples of the state simply abandoning its responsibilities to the most marginalised. The South African scandal (covered in Chapter 6) is the most recent and horrific example of this. However, there are many examples in both the US and UK where the asylum was closed and replaced by a hidden institution – a network of supported housing, poor quality bed and breakfast and homeless accommodation, as well as prisons.

In the earliest criticism of community care, it was the progressive critics of institutionalised psychiatry who were deemed most responsible for its failings. In 1982 Weismann wrote 'Foucault and the Bag Lady' about the admission of a homeless woman to Bellvue

Hospital in New York. This paper, as well as painting a very sympathetic portrait of the woman, comes to the strong conclusion that the closure of asylums led to her living on the streets. In 1982, in a debate with Foucault conducted in the book review section of the *New York Times*, the historian Lawrence Stone made a similar claim. In Torrey's (1998) view, for example, the focus on individual rights meant that services could not intervene at all. There should, in theory, be no reason why increased legal protections for patients or those being assessed under the MHA or equivalent legislation should lead to homelessness. In focusing on this side of the argument, the fiscal environment is ignored. Andrew Goldstein had been admitted to hospital on a voluntary basis on 13 occasions. He was then virtually abandoned by the therapeutic state. Christopher Clunis was legally entitled to aftercare at the time that he murdered Jonathan Zito. This in no way lessens the appalling impact of those crimes, it is rather to ask fundamental questions about the nature and structure of mental health services in the period. Any analysis that ignores the economic context will be fundamentally flawed. It seems rather unlikely that the Thatcher and Reagan governments were readers of the work of Foucault and Goffman.

If the modern period of deinstitutionalisation symbolically began with Powell's Water Tower Speech, then it ended with the introduction of CTOs in the 2007 reform of the MHA. Moves to CTOs can be traced back to the inquiries of the 1980s and 1990s. New Labour's position as outlined in *Modernising Mental Health Services* (Department of Health, 1998) was as follows:

> Although with staff dedication and commitment the policy of care in the community has benefited many, there have been too many failures. Failure has been caused by:
>
> • inadequate care, poor management of resources and underfunding;
> • the proper range of services not always being available to provide the care and support people need;
> • patients and service users not remaining in contact with services;
> • families who have willingly played a part in providing care have been overburdened;
> • problems in recruiting and retaining staff;
> • an outdated legal framework which failed to support effective treatment outside hospital.

It is important to note that the document includes underfunding as one of the key factors in what is termed – the *failure of community care*. It is, perhaps, not too surprising that the Blair administration elected with a huge majority after almost 20 years of Tory government was prepared to make such a statement. It should also be added that there then followed a period of investment in mental health services. However, within these statements one can also see clear traces of the 'pendulum has swung too far towards patients' rights' argument. This is a recurring theme in the analysis of community care – it is the legal rather than the fiscal framework that is most often seen as the cause of failure. As noted in the discussion of the introduction of Kendra's Law, it is very rare for a new legal framework to be accompanied by new resources.

Modernising Mental Health Services went on to state, among a range of reforms, that

> We will modernise mental health services by providing safe, sound and supportive services:
>
> • services should be safe, to protect the public and provide effective care for those with mental illness at the time they need it;
> • services should be sound, ensuring that patients and service users have access to the full range of services which they need;
> • services should be supportive, working with patients and service users, their families and carers to build healthier communities.

These are sentiments that are difficult to disagree with. However, it is striking that the focus of the document is on organisational issues rather than the values that underpin services. There is a focus on safety and public protection – clearly important issues. The point here is the way that they have come to dominate discussions and debates about reform. The announcement of the Wessely Review showed that the aims of *Modernising Mental Health Services* had not been achieved. In particular, two areas that have been the source of frustration in mental health services for some time – limited out of hours provision and the failure to achieve consistent service user involvement in their own care – were areas that the Wessely Review was asked to examine.

Conclusion

This volume has outlined the way that there has been a shift in the provision of mental health care. Despite commits by government of all colours to community care, a very significant proportion of mental health spending remains on institutionalised forms of care. These institutions are not the huge ones built in the 1800s. They do not have the same public profile, but the institution remains in the form of the patchwork of mental health professionals, supported housing projects, voluntary centres and groups, homelessness projects and, most regrettably, the CJS that provides some form of support to individuals experiencing mental distress. In researching this work, I have not really encountered a blueprint for community care but surely this was not what reformers had in mind. Surely, even fiscal conservatives would baulk at the cost of using the CJS as a means to access mental health care. In the UK, people with mental health problems now have legal protections against discrimination in areas such as housing and employment in a stark contrast to patients in institutions who were effectively deprived of the fundamental rights of citizenship. Progressive optimism health has been replaced by resigned fatalism. 'In crisis' has been replaced by 'at risk'.

Community care is a term that seems to have largely disappeared from public and policy discourse. For example, in establishing the Wessely Review, Theresa May focused on the use of the MHA rather than the broader issues that face mental health services. The 'disappearance' of community care from debates might reflect that its basic premises are now deeply engrained and widely accepted. The asylums have disappeared literally and metaphorically. There is thus no need to make the case for community-based mental health provision. This is an optimistic reading – an alternative is that a form of therapeutic pessimism has come to dominate mental health policy. The closure of the asylums has not altered the fact that the majority of limited mental health budgets are spent on institutional care. In fact, one of the major and most consistently highlighted concerns in mental health services is *the lack of mental health beds* rather than *the lack of alternatives to mental health beds*.

Simon and Rosenbaum (2015) note that mental health policy is cyclical, characterised by periods of boom and bust. There are periods where the fundamental questions of how society should respond to citizens who experience mental distress make their way to the top of the social policy agenda. This usually follows an institutional scandal of some sort. There then follows a period where these questions are debated, an Inquiry or Commission may be established, reforms to legislation are recommended, new policies or ways of working are introduced. There may even be a period of increased investment in services and attempts to change social attitudes. These issues then retreat from the public view, replaced by another social welfare issue – often involving responses to child abuse and neglect. The policy of deinstitutionalisation was the result of a period when the institution of the mental health hospital came under huge criticism. The asylum was presented as a Gothic abusive institution essentially beyond reform. These attacks were based on the abusive practices that existed in the asylums. In addition, critics such as Basaglia and Goffman mounted an ideological opposition to these institutions that they, correctly in my view, saw as denying those who were incarcerated in them fundamental human rights.

There was a coming together of the right and the left. Fiscal conservatives concerned about the extent of state provision on welfare generally saw the asylum regime as a drain on the public purse. The libertarian right, mostly clearly in the figure of Szasz, saw the psychiatric system as an example of overmighty interference in the lives of citizens. The combination of fiscal conservatism and strands of radicalism progressive ideas is evident in Enoch Powell's Water Tower speech. Powell, an ideological inspiration to Thatcherism was, possibly, as far removed from the Gramscian intellectual Basaglia as it was possible to be. His speech mentions progress in treatment, but economic concerns are never far from the surface. The result of this mixing of the right and left was that in the early 1960s, there were few voices that opposed the policy of deinstitutionalisation. Shen and Snowden (2014), in their analysis of the impact of deinstitutionalisation, highlight how widespread the policy has become. They examine its impact in 190 countries. It is a policy that has the support of the World Health Organisation. They note that it has become something of a marker of 'progress'. Moves away from institutionalised forms of care are apparent in other areas such as learning disability services. They argue that these changes are often introduced in a wave of optimism with little consideration of the local conditions. Deinstitutionalisation is a mark of modernity and transition, possibly linked to wider political changes such as the establishment of liberal democracy and strengthening the institutions of civil society. The South African scandal shows that there are dangers in this headlong rush to reform.

In 1979, in an article in *Hospital and Community Psychiatry*, Talbot (2004), in reviewing what he saw as the disastrous failure of deinstitutionalisation, ended the piece with what he termed his Ten Commandments – the lessons learnt from deinstitutionalization:

- Before patients are discharged, there must be an adequate number and range of community services and facilities to provide patients with treatment, care, and community support.
- Barriers to full participation in health and mental health delivery systems must be removed so that existing eligibility and reimbursement practices that discriminate against the chronically mentally ill are not perpetuated.
- Chronically mentally ill patients must have full civil rights and opportunities, including equal access to housing, education, vocational rehabilitation, income maintenance, and adequate care in the community.
- Money must follow patients. That is, funding must be as flexible as patient populations, and if there are further shifts in the locations of care or treatment, monies must accompany the patients to meet their needs.
- Medical–psychiatric money should be separate from but coordinated with funding for community support (for example, housing, food, income support, social services, and vocational and social rehabilitation). It is especially critical to keep this requirement in mind when considering what benefits are to be included under national health insurance.
- A system that ensures continuity of care must be developed. To date, the degree of achievement of this truism is inversely related to its utterance.
- A case management system must be established. Such a system should not create a whole new profession or paraprofession but should make use of existing manpower and resources.
- Services should be provided by the smallest local entity that is capable of delivering such services. Such entities must designate a specific person or facility as the core service agency of the service delivery system.
- Federal, state, and local governments should divest themselves of the conflict of interest inherent in both contracting for services and operating services themselves. If local entities operate services, city and county governments can monitor and plan them on

their level, states can coordinate a statewide plan, and the federal government can oversee a national effort.

There must be a concerted national effort that would increase and continue existing research into the causes of chronicity, its prevention, effective treatment, and model service systems for the chronically ill.

Reading them 40 years on, it is shocking how relevant they remain. On one level, it seems odd that there remains a need to make the moral case for community care. The fiscal case was, not surprisingly, quickly accepted by governments committed to reducing welfare spending and the role of the social state. The progressive argument for community care was not about cost cutting, it was about critical perspectives on the exercise of power, social investment, human rights and dignity; ideas that should never lose their strength and relevance. The 'new case' for community care is not a reboot. It will involve exploring new approaches to the causes of mental illness. It will also require shifts in the entrenched power of mental health professionals alongside dynamic, progressive ways of working. It is only be learning from the failures of the past that a repeat of them can be avoided. The basis of the new community care needs to be a revitalised and reinvigorated value base with the concept of dignity at its core.

References

Adebowale, Lord (2013) *Independent Commission on Mental Health and Policing Report*, Independent Commission on Mental Health and Policing.

Alexander, M. (2012) *The New Jim Crow: Mass Incarceration in the Age of Colorblindness*, New York: New Press.

Alston, P. (2018) *Statement on Visit to the United Kingdom, by Professor Philip Alston, United Nations Special Rapporteur on Extreme Poverty and Human Rights*, 16 November, www.ohchr.org/Documents/Issues/ Poverty EOM_GB_16Nov2018.pdf

Altamura, A.C. and Goodwin, G.M. (2010) 'How Law 180 in Italy has reshaped psychiatry after 30 years: past attitudes, current trends and unmet needs', *The British Journal of Psychiatry*, 197(4): 261–2.

Amador, X.F. (2006) *Poor Insight in Schizophrenia: An Overview and Impact on Medication and Compliance*, New York: McMohan Publishing Group.

Anderson, B. (2006) *Imagined Communities: Reflections on the Origin and Spread of Nationalism*, London: Verso Books.

Antonakakis, N. and Collins, A. (2016) 'The impact of fiscal austerity on suicide mortality: Evidence across the "Eurozone periphery"', *Social Science and Medicine*, 145: 63–78.

Applebaum, P.S. (2005) 'Law & Psychiatry: Assessing Kendra's Law: Five Years of Outpatient Commitment in New York', *Psychiatric Services*, 56(7): 791–2.

Arendt, H. (1959) *The Human Condition: A Study of the Central Dilemmas Facing Modern Man*, New York: Doubleday.

Arendt, H. (1973) *The Origins of Totalitarianism*, New York: Houghton Mifflin Harcourt.

Audit Commission for Local Authorities and the National Health Service in England and Wales (1994) *Finding a Place: A Review of Mental Health Services for Adults*, HM Stationery Office.

Banongo, E., Davies, J. and Godin, P. (2005) *Engaging Service Users in the Evaluation and Development of Forensic Mental Health Care Service*, London: City University Media Development Unit.

Barnes, D., Carpenter, J. and Dickinson, C. (2006) 'The outcomes of partnerships with mental health service users in interprofessional education: a case study', *Health & Social Care in the Community*, *14*(5): 426–435.

Barnes, M. and Prior, D. (2009) 'Examining the idea of 'subversion' in public services', in M. Barnes and D. Prior (eds), *Subversive Citizens: Power, Agency and Resistance in Public Services*, Bristol: Policy Press, pp 3–16.

Barr, B., Taylor-Robinson, D., Stuckler, D., Loopstra, R., Reeves, A. and Whitehead, M. (2016) ' "First do no harm": Are disability assessments associated with adverse trends in mental health? A longitudinal study', *Journal of Epidemiology & Community Health*, 70: 339–45.

Barr, H. (2001) 'Policing madness: people with mental illness and the NYPD', in A. McArdle and T. Erzen (eds), *Zero Tolerance: Quality of Life and the New Police Brutality in New York City*, New York: NYU Press, pp 50–84.

Bartlett, A. and Hollins, S. (2018) 'Challenges and mental health needs of women in prison', *The British Journal of Psychiatry*, 212(3): 134–136.

Barton, W.R. (1959) *Institutional Neurosis*, Bristol: Wright and Sons.

Basaglia, F. (1968) *L'Istituzione negata*, Torino: Einaudi.

Bauman, Z. (2001) *Community: Seeking Safety in an Insecure World*, Cambridge: Polity Press.

Bauman, Z. (2007) *Liquid Modernity: Living in an Age of Uncertainty*, Cambridge: Polity Press.

BBC News (1998) 'Care in the community to be scrapped', 17 January, http://news.bbc.co.uk/1/hi/uk/48168.stm

BBC News (2019) 'Mental Health: police detentions up 30% in five years', 30 October, https://www.bbc.co.uk/news/uk-wales-50222385

Beatty, C. and Fothergill, S. (2016) *The Uneven Impact of Welfare Reform: The Financial Losses to Places and People*, project report, Sheffield: Centre for Regional Economic and Social Research.

Bebbington, P., Jakobowitz, S., McKenzie, N., Killaspy, H., Iveson, R., Duffield, G. and Kerr, M. (2017) 'Assessing needs for psychiatric treatment in prisoners: 1. Prevalence of disorder', *Social psychiatry and psychiatric epidemiology*, *52*(2): 221–229.

Beck, U. (1992) *Risk Society: Towards a New Modernity* (translated by M. Ritter), London: Sage.

Becker, G.S. (1968) 'Crime and punishment: An economic approach', in N.G. Fielding, A. Clarke and R. Witt (eds), *The Economic Dimensions of Crime*, London: Palgrave Macmillan, pp 13–68.

Berman, G. (2012) *Prison Population Statistics*, House of Commons Library.

Bhui, K., Stansfeld, S., Hull, S., Mole, F. and Feder, G. (2003) 'Ethnic variations in pathways to and use of specialist mental health services in the UK. Systematic review', *British Journal of Psychiatry*, 182: 105–16.

Birmingham, L. (2003) 'The mental health of prisoners', *Advances in Psychiatric Treatment*, 9(3): 191–9.

Birmingham, L. (2004) 'Mental disorder and prisons', *Psychiatric Bulletin*, 28(11): 393–7.

Bittner, E. (1967) 'The police on skid-row: A study of peace keeping', *American Sociological Review*, 32(5): 699–715.

Bittner, E. (1970) *The Functions of the Police in Modern Society*, Volume 88, Chevy Chase, MD: National Institute of Mental Health.

Blofeld, J. (2004) *Independent Inquiry into the Death of David Bennett*, Cambridge: Norfolk, Suffolk and Cambridgeshire Strategic Health Authority.

Blom-Cooper, L. (1985) *A Child in Trust: The Report of the Panel of Inquiry into the Circumstances Surrounding the Death of Jasmine Beckford*, London: London Borough of Brent.

Blom-Cooper, L., Hally, H. and Murphy, E. (1995) *The Falling Shadow: One Patient's Mental Health Care, 1978–1993*, London: Duckworth.

Blom-Cooper, L. (1999) 'Public Inquiries in mental health (with particular reference to the Blackwood case at Broadmoor and the patient-complaints of Ashworth Hospital)', in D. Webb and R. Harris (eds), *Mentally Disordered Offenders*, London: Routledge, pp 27–37.

Booth, W. (1890) *In Darkest England and the Way Out*, London: International Headquarters of the Salvation Army.

Borschmann, R.D., Gillard, S., Turner, K., Lovell, K., Goodrich-Purnell, N. and Chambers, M. (2010) 'Demographic and referral patterns of people detained under Section 136 of the Mental Health Act (1983) in a south London Mental Health Trust from 2005 to 2008', *Medicine, Science and the Law*, 50(1): 15–18.

Bourdieu, P. (1998) 'The left hand and the right hand of the state', in P. Bourdieu (ed), *Acts of resistance: Against the tyranny of the market*, New York: New Press, pp 1–10.

Bourdieu, P. et al (1999) *The Weight of the World: Social Suffering in Contemporary Society*, Cambridge: Polity Press

Bourdieu, P. (2001) *Acts of Resistance*, Cambridge: Polity Press.

Bowcott, O. and Duncan, P. (2018) 'Strain of legal cuts shows in family, housing and immigration courts', *The Guardian*, 26 December, www.theguardian.com/law/2018/dec/26/strain-of-legal-aid-cuts-showing-in-family-housing-and-immigration-law

Bradley, K.J.C.B. (2008). *The Bradley Report: Lord Bradley's Review of People with Mental Health Problems or Learning Disabilities in the Criminal Justice System*, Volume 7, London: Department of Health.

Brenner, N. and Theodore, N. (2002) 'Cities and the geographies of "actually existing neoliberalism"', *Antipode*, 34(3): 349–79.

Brown, W. (2015) *Undoing the Demos: Neoliberalism's Stealth Revolution*, Cambridge, MA: MIT Press.

Bunting, M. (2003) 'Passion and pessimism', *The Guardian*, 5 April, www.theguardian.com/books/2003/apr/05/society

Butler, I. and Drakeford, M. (2005) *Scandal, Social Policy and Social Welfare*, Bristol: Policy Press.

Cameron, D. (2015) 'My vision for a smarter state', speech, 11 September, www.gov.uk/government/speeches/prime-minister-my-vision-for-a-smarter-state

Care Quality Commission (2018) 'Monitoring the Mental Health Act Report', www.cqc.org.uk/publications/major-report/monitoring-mental-health-act-report

Carey, J. (2012) *The Intellectuals and the Masses: Pride and Prejudice among the Literary Intelligentsia 1880–1939*, London: Faber & Faber.

Carey, S.J. (2001) 'Police officers' knowledge of, and attitudes towards, mental illness in southwest Scotland', *Scottish Medical Journal*, 46(2): 41–2.

Carson, E. and Golinelli, D. (2013) *Prisoners in 2012: Trends in Admissions and Releases 1991–2013*, U.S. Department of Justice, www.bjs.gov/content/pub/pdf/p12tar9112.pdf

Castel, R. (1988) *The Regulation of Madness*, Cambridge: Polity Press.

Cavadino, M. and Dignan, J. (with others) (2006) *Penal Systems: A Comparative Approach*, London: Sage.

Centre for Mental Health (2008) *Briefing 36: Police and mental health,* London: Centre for Mental Health.

Centre for Welfare Reform (2015) 'A Fair Society: Centre for Welfare Reform', www.centreforwelfarereform.org

Chambers, M. (2005) 'A concept analysis of therapeutic relationships', in J. Cutcliffe and H. McKenna (eds), *The Essential Concepts of Nursing*, Edinburgh: Elsevier, pp 301–16.

Chaplin, R. and Peters, S. (2003) 'Executives have taken over the asylum: the fate of 71 psychiatric hospitals', *Psychiatric Bulletin*, 27(6): 227–9.

Clare, A. (2012) *Psychiatry in Dissent: Controversial issues in thought and practice* (2nd edn), London: Routledge.

Clarke, J. and Newman, J. (2012) 'The alchemy of austerity', *Critical Social Policy*, 32(3): 299–319.

Clear, T. (2009) *Imprisoning Communities: How Mass Incarceration Makes Disadvantaged Neighborhoods Worse*, New York: Oxford University Press.

Cohen, S. (1972) *Folk Devils and Moral Panics*, London: Macgibbon and Kee.

Cohen, S. (2011) 'Whose side were we on? The undeclared politics of moral panic theory', *Crime, Media, Culture*, 7(3): 237–43.

Coid, J.W. (1994) 'The Christopher Clunis enquiry', *Psychiatric Bulletin*, 18(8): 449–52.

Community Consortium (2015) 'The Willard Suitcases', The Lives They Left Behind: Suitcases from a State Hospital Attic, www.suitcaseexhibit.org/index.php?section=about&subsection=suitcases

Cooper, G. (1998) 'Schizophrenic visited clinic before killing', *The Independent*, 14 November, www.independent.co.uk/news/schizophrenic-visited-clinic-before-killing-1184675.html

Cooper, V. and Whyte, D. (2017) *The Violence of Austerity*, London: Pluto Press.

Coppock, V. and Hopton, J. (2002) *Critical Perspectives on Mental Health*, London: Routledge.

Corston, J. (2007) *The Corston Report: A Report by Baroness Jean Corston of a Review of Women with Particular Vulnerabilities in the Criminal Justice System*, London: Home Office.

Crichton, J.H. (2011) 'A review of published independent inquiries in England into psychiatric patient homicide, 1995–2010', *Journal of Forensic Psychiatry & Psychology*, 22(6): 761–89.

Cross, S. (2010) *Mediating Madness: Mental Distress and Cultural Representation*, Basingstoke: Palgrave Macmillan.

Crossley, S. (2016) '"Realising the (troubled) family", "crafting the neoliberal state"'. *Families, Relationships and Societies*, 5(2): 263–79.

Crow, G.P. and Allan, G. (1995) 'Community types, community typologies and community time', *Time & Society*, 4(2): 147–66.

Cummins, I. (2006) 'A path not taken? Mentally disordered offenders and the criminal justice system', *Journal of Social Welfare and Family Law*, 28(3–4): 267–81.

Cummins, I. (2010a) 'Deinstitutionalisation: mental health services in the age of neo-liberalism', *Social Policy and Social Work in Transition*, 1(2): 55–74.

Cummins, I. (2010b) 'Distant voices, still lives: reflections on the impact of media reporting of the cases of Christopher Clunis and Ben Silcock', *Ethnicity and Inequalities in Health and Social Care*, 3(4): 18–29.

Cummins, I. (2012) 'Using Simon's Governing through crime to explore the development of mental health policy in England and Wales since 1983', *Journal of Social Welfare and Family Law*, 34(3): 325–37.

Cummins, I. (2015) 'Discussing race, racism and mental health: two mental health inquiries reconsidered', *International Journal of Human Rights in Healthcare*, 8(3): 160–72.

Cummins, I. (2016) *Mental Health and the Criminal Justice System: A social work perspective*, Northwich: Critical Publishing.

Cummins, I. (2017a) *Critical Psychiatry: A Biography*, Northwich: Critical Publishing.

Cummins, I. (2017b) 'From hero of the counterculture to risk assessment: a consideration of two portrayals of the "psychiatric patient"', *Illness, Crisis & Loss*, 26(2): 111–23.

Cummins, I. (2018a) *Poverty, Inequality and Social Work: The Impact of Neo-liberalism and Austerity Politics on Welfare Provision*, Bristol: Policy Press.

Cummins, I. (2018b) 'The impact of austerity on mental health service provision: A UK perspective', *International Journal of Environmental Research and Public Health*, 15(6): 1145.

Cummins, I. (2019) *Mental Health Social Work Reimagined*, Bristol: Policy Press.

Cummins, I. and Edmondson, D. (2016) 'Policing and street triage', *The Journal of Adult Protection*, 18(1): 40–52.

Cummins, I., Foley, M. and King, M. (2014) '"… And after the break": police officers' views of TV crime drama', *Policing: A Journal of Policy and Practice*, 8(2): 205–11.

Davis, M. (1998) *City of Quartz: Excavating the Future in Los Angeles*, New York: Vintage.

Dawson, J. and Romans, S. (2001) 'Uses of community treatment orders in New Zealand: early findings', *Australian & New Zealand Journal of Psychiatry*, 35(2): 190–195.

Department of Health (1992) *Report of the Committee of Inquiry into Complaints about Ashworth Hospital* (Chairman: Sir Louis Blom-Cooper QC), London: HMSO.

Department of Health (1994) 'Guidance on the discharge of mentally disordered people and their continuing care in the community', HSG (94)27, 10 May, London: Department of Health.

Department of Health (1995) *The Mental Health (Patients in the Community) Act*, London: HMSO.

Department of Health (1998) *Modernising Mental Health Services: Safe, Sound and Supportive*, London: HMSO.

Department of Health (2006) *Our Health, Our Care, Our Say: A New Direction for Community Services*, London: HMSO.

Department of Health and Social Care (2018) *Modernising the Mental Health Act: Final Report from the Independent Review* (Chairman: Professor Sir Simon Wessely), www.gov.uk/government/publications/modernising-the-mental-health-act-final-report-from-the-independent-review

DHSS (1988) *Report of the Committee of Inquiry into the Care and Aftercare of Sharon Campbell* (Chairman: John Spokes), London: HMSO.

Downes, D. and Hansen, K. (2006) 'Welfare and Punishment: The Relationship between Welfare Spending and Imprisonment', London: Crime and Society Foundation, www.crimeandsociety.org.uk

Drucker, E. (2011) *A Plagues of Prisons: The Epidemiology of Mass Incarceration in America*, New York: New Press.

Dunn, B. (2017) 'Against neoliberalism as a concept', *Capital & Class*, 41(3): 435–54.

Dunn, J. and Fahy, T.A. (1990) 'Police admissions to a psychiatric hospital: demographic and clinical differences between ethnic groups', *The British Journal of Psychiatry*, 156(3): 373–8.

Dworkin, R. (1995) *Life's Dominion*, London: HarperCollins.

Eastman, N. (1994) 'Mental health law: civil liberties and the principle of reciprocity', *BMJ*, 308(6920): 43.

Eastman, N. and Starling, B. (2006) 'Mental disorder ethics: theory and empirical investigation', *Journal of Medical Ethics*, 32: 94–9.

Eaton, W. (1980) 'A formal theory of selection for schizophrenia', *American Journal of Sociology*, 86: 149–58.

Emejulu, A. and Bassel, L. (2015) 'Minority women, austerity and activism', *Race & Class*, 57(2): 86–95.

Estroff, S.E. (1981) 'Psychiatric deinstitutionalization: A sociocultural analysis', *Journal of Social Issues*, 37(3): 116–32.

Faraone, S. (1982) 'Psychiatry and political repression in the Soviet Union', *American Psychologist*, 37(10): 1105–12.

Fallon, P., Bluglass, R., Edwards, B. and Daniels, G. (1999) *Report of the Committee of Inquiry into the Personality Disorder Unit, Ashworth Special Hospital*, London: Stationery Office.

Fanon, F. (2008) *Black Skin, White Masks*, New York: Grove Press.

Farnham, F.R. and James, D.V. (2000) 'Patients' attitudes to psychiatric hospital admission', *The Lancet*, 355(9204): 594.

Faulkner, A. (1997) *Knowing Our Own Minds*, London: Mental Health Foundation.

Fazel, S. and Seewald, K. (2012) 'Severe mental illness in 33 588 prisoners worldwide: systematic review and meta-regression analysis', *The British Journal of Psychiatry*, 200(5): 364–373.

Fazel, S., Grann, M., Kling, B. and Hawton, K. (2011) 'Prison suicide in 12 countries: An ecological study of 861 suicides during 2003–2007', *Social Psychiatry and Psychiatric Epidemiology*, 46 (3): 191–195

Fazel, S., Hayes, A.J., Bartellas, K., Clerici, M. and Trestman, R. (2016) 'Mental health of prisoners: prevalence, adverse outcomes, and interventions', *The Lancet Psychiatry*, 3(9): 871–881.

Fazel, S., Ramesh, T. and Hawton, K. (2017) 'Suicide in prisons: an international study of prevalence and contributory factors', *The Lancet Psychiatry*, 4(12): 946–952.

Fendler, L. (2004) 'Praxis and agency in Foucault's historiography', *Studies in Philosophy and Education*, 23(5–6): 445–66.

Fennell, P. (2002) *Treatment Without Consent: Law, Psychiatry and the Treatment of Mentally Disordered People Since 1845*, London: Routledge.

Fineman, M. (2004) *The Autonomy Myth: A Theory of Dependency*, New York: The New Press.

Foot, J. (2015) *The Man who Closed the Asylums: Franco Basaglia and the Revolution in Mental Health Care*, London: Verso Books.

Foucault, M. (1982) 'The subject and power', *Critical Inquiry*, 8(4): 777–95.

Foucault, M. (2003) *Madness and Civilization*, London: Routledge.

Foucault, M. (2008) *The Birth of Biopolitics: Lectures at the Collège de France 1978–1979*, Basingstoke: Palgrave Macmillan.

Foucault, M. (2012) *Discipline and Punish: The Birth of the Prison*, London: Vintage.

Franklin, B. (2002) 'Hospital-heritage-home: Reconstructing the nineteenth century lunatic asylum', *Housing, Theory and Society*, 19(3–4): 170–84.

Fraser, N. (2017) 'The end of progressive neoliberalism', *Dissent*, 2 January, www.dissentmagazine.org/online_articles/progressive-neoliberalism-reactionary-populism-nancy-fraser

Friedman, M. (2009) *Capitalism and Freedom* (49th anniversary edn), London: University of Chicago Press.

Garland, D. (2001) *The Culture of Control*, Oxford: Oxford University Press.

Garland, D. (2004) 'Beyond the culture of control', *Critical Review of International Social and Political Philosophy* (Special issue on Garland's *The Culture of Control*), 7(2): 160–89.

Garland, D. (2014) *What is the Welfare State? A Sociological Restatement*, available at https://youtu.be/n0zkOFzkpeY

Garrett, P. (2017) *Welfare Words: Critical Social Work & Social Policy*, London: Sage.

Garrett, P.M. (2007) 'Making social work more Bourdieusian: Why the social professions should critically engage with the work of Pierre Bourdieu', *European Journal of Social Work*, 10(2): 225–43.

Garrett, P.M. (2018) 'Revisiting "The Birth of Biopolitics": Foucault's account of neoliberalism and the remaking of social policy', *Journal of Social Policy*, 48(3): 469–487.

Giddens, A. (1991) *Modernity and self-identity: Self and society in the late modern age*, Stanford: Stanford University Press.

Giroux, H. (2011) 'Neoliberalism and the death of the social state: Remembering Walter Benjamin's Angel of History Social Identities', *Journal for the Study of Race, Nation and Culture*, 17(4): 587–601.

Goffman, E. (1969) 'The insanity of place', *Psychiatry*, 32(4): 357–88.

Goffman, E. (2014) *Asylums: Essays on the Social Situation of Mental Patients and Other Inmates*, London: Routledge.

Goodman, P.S. (2018) 'In Britain, austerity is changing everything', *New York Times*, 28 May, www.nytimes.com/2018/05/28/world/europe/uk-austerity-poverty.html

Google Play (no date) 'Adventure Escape: Asylum', https://play.google.com/store/apps/details?id=com.haikugamesco.escapeasylum&hl=en_GB

Gostin, L.O. (2007) 'From a civil libertarian to a sanitarian', *Journal of Law and Society*, 34(4): 594–616.

Gostin, L.O. (2012) 'A framework convention on global health: health for all, justice for all', *JAMA*, 307(19): 2087–92.

Gottschalk, M. (2006) *The Prison and the Gallows: The Politics of Mass Incarceration in America*, Cambridge: Cambridge University Press.

Green, E. (2016) 'What are the most-cited publications in the social sciences (according to Google Scholar)?', LSE Impact Blog, 12 May, https://blogs.lse.ac.uk/impactofsocialsciences/2016/05/12/what-are-the-most-cited-publications-in-the-social-sciences-according-to-google-scholar/

Greenwood, G. (2017) 'Police handling a third more mental health cases, figures suggest', *BBC News*, 28 October, www.bbc.co.uk/news/uk-41688577

Griffiths, R. (1988) *Community Care: Agenda for Action. A Report to the Secretary of State for Social Services*, London: HMSO.

Grover, C. (2018) 'Violent proletarianisation: Social murder, the reserve army of labour and social security "austerity" in Britain', *Critical Social Policy*, 39(3): 335–355.

Guardian (2012) 'George Osborne tells Tory conference: 'We're all in this together' – video', available at www.theguardian.com/politics/video/2012/oct/08/george-osborne-tory-conference-video

Gunn, J. (2000) 'Future directions for treatment in forensic psychiatry', *British Journal of Psychiatry*, 176: 332–8.

Habermas, J. (2010) 'The concept of human dignity and the realistic utopia of human rights', *Metaphilosophy*, 41(4): 468–80.

Hall, S. (1979) 'The Great Moving Right Show', *Marxism Today*, January: 14–20.

Hall, S., Critcher, C., Jefferson, T., Clarke, J. and Roberts, B. (2013) *Policing the Crisis: Mugging, The State and Law and Order*, London: Palgrave Macmillan.

Harcourt, B.E. (2005) 'From the asylum to the prison: Rethinking the incarceration revolution', *Texas Law Review*, 84: 1751.

Harcourt, B.E. (2010) 'Risk as a Proxy for Race', University of Chicago Public Law & Legal Theory Working Paper No. 323.

Harcourt, B.E. (2011) 'Reducing mass incarceration: Lessons from the deinstitutionalization of mental hospitals in the 1960s', *Ohio State Journal of Criminal Law*, 9: 53.

Harcourt, B.E. (2015) 'Risk as a proxy for race: The dangers of risk assessment', *Federal Sentencing Reporter*, 27(4): 237–243.

Harvey, D. (1990) 'Between space and time: reflections on the geographical imagination', *Annals of the Association of American Geographers*, 80(3): 418–34.

Harvey, D. (2005) *A Brief History of Neoliberalism*, Oxford: Oxford University Press.

Hatzenbuehler, M., Phelan, J. and Link, B. (2013) 'Stigma as a fundamental cause of population health inequalities', *American Journal of Public Health*, 103: 813–21.

Hawkins, S.A. and Hastie, R. (1990) 'Hindsight: Biased judgments of past events after the outcomes are known', *Psychological Bulletin*, 107(3): 311.

Hay, C. (1995) 'Mobilization through interpellation: James Bulger, juvenile crime and the construction of a moral panic', *Social & Legal Studies*, 4(2): 197–223.

Hayek, F.A. (2014) *The road to serfdom: Text and documents: The definitive edition*, London: Routledge.

Her Majesty's Inspectorate of Prisons for England and Wales (HMIP) (2017) *Annual Report 2016–17*, HC 208, 18 July, www.justiceinspectorates.gov.uk/hmiprisons/wpcontent/uploads/sites/4/2017/07/HMIP-AR_2016-17_CONTENT_201017_WEB.pdf

HMIP (2018) *Annual Report 2017–18*, HC 1245, 11 July, www.justiceinspectorates.gov.uk/hmiprisons/wp-content/uploads/sites/4/2018/07/6.5053_HMI-Prisons_AR-2017-18_revised_web.pdf

Hilton, C. (2007) 'Changes between the 1959 and 1983 Mental Health Acts (England & Wales), with particular reference to consent to treatment for electroconvulsive therapy', *History of Psychiatry*, 18(2): 217–29.

Hirsch, S. (2018) *In the Shadow of Enoch Powell: Race, Locality and Resistance*, Manchester: Manchester University Press.

Hoggett, B. (1984) *Mental Health Law*, London: Sweet & Maxwell

Home Affairs Select Committee (2015) *Policing and mental health: Eleventh report of session 2014–15*, London: The Stationery Office Limited.

House of Commons (1990) *The National Health Service and Community Care Act*, London: HMSO.

House of Commons Home Affairs Select Committee (2018) *Policing for the Future*, HC 515, 25 October, https://publications.parliament. uk/pa/cm201719/cmselect/cmhaff/515/515.pdf

Howard, E. (2018) 'The end of Italy's asylums', Magnum Photos, 12 May, www.magnumphotos.com/arts-culture/society-arts-culture/ raymond-depardon-end-italys-asylums

Howard, J. (1780) *The State of the Prisons in England and Wales*, W. Eyres.

Howe, G. (1969) *Report of the Committee of Inquiry into Allegations of Ill-Treatment of Patients and other irregularities at the Ely Hospital*, Cm 3975, Cardiff.

Hutton, W. (1996) *The State We're In*, London: Random House.

Ignatieff, M. (1985) 'State, civil society and total institutions', in S. Cohen and A. Scull (eds), *Social Control and the State: Historical and Comparative Essays*, Oxford: Blackwell.

Ingleby, D. (1980) *Critical Psychiatry: The Politics of Mental Health*, London: Free Association Books.

Jensen, T. and Tyler, I. (2015) '"Benefits broods": The cultural and political crafting of anti-welfare common sense', *Critical Social Policy*, 35(4): 1–22.

Jones, K. (1960) *Mental Health and Social Policy, 1845–1959*, London: Routledge and Kegan Paul.

Jones, R. (2014) *The Story of Baby P: Setting the Record Straight*, Bristol: Policy Press.

Jones, S.L. and Mason, T. (2002) 'Quality of treatment following police detention of mentally disordered offenders', *Journal of Psychiatric and Mental Health Nursing*, 9(1): 73–80.

Joseph, A.E. and Kearns, R.A. (1996) 'Deinstitutionalization meets restructuring: the closure of a psychiatric hospital in New Zealand', *Health & Place*, 2(3): 179–89.

Kant, I. (1996) *The Metaphysics of Morals* (edited and translated by Mary J. Gregor), Cambridge: Cambridge University Press.

Karban, K. (2016) 'Developing a health inequalities approach for mental health social work', *British Journal of Social Work*, 47: 885–992.

Keïteï (2011) 'West Park Asylum', The Urban Adventures of Keïteï – Explore Everything, 3 February, http://keiteisurbanadventures. blogspot.com/2011/03/west-park-espom-february-2011.html

Kelly, B. (2007) 'Penrose's Law in Ireland: an ecological analysis of psychiatric inpatients and prisoners', *Irish Medical Journal*, 100: 373–4.

Keown, P., Murphy, H., McKenna, D. and McKinnon, I. (2018) 'Changes in the use of the Mental Health Act 1983 in England 1984/ 85 to 2015/16', *The British Journal of Psychiatry*, 213(4): 595–9.

Kesey, K. (1962) *One Flew Over the Cuckoo's Nest*, London: Penguin.

Knowles, C. (2000) *Bedlam on the Streets*, London: Routledge.

Kynaston, D. (2008) *Austerity Britain, 1945–1951*, Volume 1, London: A&C Black.

Lacey, N. (2008) *The Prisoners' Dilemma: Political Economy and Punishment in Contemporary Democracies*, Cambridge: Cambridge University Press.

Laing, J.M. (2000) 'Rights versus risk? Reform of the Mental Health Act 1983', *Medical Law Review*, 8(2): 210–50.

Laing, R. (1959) *The Divided Self*, London: Tavistock.

Laing, R. (1967) *The Politics of Experience and the Bird of Paradise*, Harmondsworth: Penguin.

Lammy, D. (2017) *The Lammy Review: An Independent Review into the Treatment of, and Outcomes for, Black, Asian and Minority Ethnic Individuals in the Criminal Justice System*, HM Government.

Large, M., Smith, G., Swinson, N., Shaw, J. and Nielssen, O. (2008) 'Homicide due to mental disorder in England and Wales over 50 years', *The British Journal of Psychiatry*, 193(2): 130–3.

Large, M.M. and Nielssen, O. (2009) 'The Penrose hypothesis in 2004: Patient and prisoner numbers are positively correlated in low-and-middle income countries but are unrelated in high-income countries', *Psychology and Psychotherapy: Theory, Research and Practice*, 82(1): 113–19.

Lawton-Smith, S., Dawson, J. and Burns, T. (2008) 'Community treatment orders are not a good thing', *The British Journal of Psychiatry*, 193(2): 96–100.

Leary, J.P. (2011) 'Detroitism: What does "ruin porn" tell us about the motor city?', *Guernica*, 15 January, www.guernicamag.com/leary_ 1_15_11/

Leff, J. (ed) (1997) *Care in the Community: Illusion or Reality*, London: Wiley.

Leff, J. and Trieman, N. (2000) 'Long-stay patients discharged from psychiatric hospital', *British Journal of Psychiatry*, 176: 217–23.

Lehane, D. (2003) *Shutter Island*, New York: HarperCollins.

Lipkin, R.J. (1990) 'Free will, responsibility and the promise of forensic psychiatry', *International Journal of Law and Psychiatry*, 13(4): 331–59.

Lipsky, M. (2010) *Street-level Bureaucracy: Dilemmas of the Individual in Public Service*, New York: Russell Sage Foundation.

López, T.M. (2014) *The Winter of Discontent: Myth, Memory, and History*, Oxford: Oxford University Press.

Lurigio, A.J. and Watson, A.C. (2010) 'The police and people with mental illness: New approaches to a longstanding problem', *Journal of Police Crisis Negotiations*, 10(1–2): 3–14.

MacCabe, C. and Yanacek, H. (eds) (2018) *Keywords for Today: A 21st Century Vocabulary*, Oxford: Oxford University Press.

Macintyre, A., Ferris, D., Gonçalves, B. and Quinn, N. (2018) 'What has economics got to do with it? The impact of socioeconomic factors on mental health and the case for collective action', *Palgrave Communications*, 4, article 10.

Maden, A. (2007) 'England's new Mental Health Act represents law catching up with science', *Philosophy, Ethics, and Humanities in Medicine*, 2: 16.

Makgoba, M.W. (2016) *The Report into the 'Circumstances Surrounding the Deaths of Mentally Ill Patients: Gauteng Province'. No Guns: 94+ Violent Deaths and Still Counting*, Office of the Health Ombud, South Africa, www.sahrc.org.za/home/21/files/Esidimeni%20full%20report.pdf

Marmot, M. (2010) *Fair Society, Healthy Lives, The Marmot Review*, London: Department of Health, www.parliament.uk/documents/fair-society-healthy-lives-full-report.pdf

Marmot, M. (2015) 'The health gap: the challenge of an unequal world', *The Lancet*, 386(10011): 2442–4.

Martin, J.P. (1985) *Hospitals in Trouble*, Oxford: Blackwell.

Mauer, M. (2006) *The Race to Incarcerate*, New York: New Press.

Mckenzie, L. (2015) *Getting By Estates, Class and Culture in Austerity Britain*, Bristol: Policy Press.

McKittrick, D. and McVea, D. (2001) *Making Sense of the Troubles: A History of the Northern Ireland Conflict*, London: Penguin.

Metzl, J.M. (2010) *The Protest Psychosis: How Schizophrenia Became a Black Disease*, Boston, MA: Beacon Press.

Mills, C. (2018) '"Dead people don't claim": A psychopolitical autopsy of UK austerity suicides', *Critical Social Policy*, 38(2): 302–22.

Mngadi, M. (2017) 'Suspended health department head to challenge Life Esidimeni arbitration subpoena', www.news24.com/SouthAfrica/News/suspended-health-department-head-to-challenge-life-esidimeni-arbitration-subpoena-20171129

Moon, G. (2000) 'Risk and protection: the discourse of confinement in contemporary mental health policy', *Health & Place*, 6(3): 239–50.

Morriss, L. (2016a) 'Being seconded to a Mental Health Trust: the (in)visibility of mental health social work', *The British Journal of Social Work*, 47(5): 1344–60.

Morriss, L. (2016b) 'AMHP work: dirty or prestigious? Dirty work designations and the approved mental health professional', *The British Journal of Social Work*, 46(3): 703–18.

Morse, S.J. (2003) 'Diminished rationality, diminished responsibility', *Ohio State Journal of Criminal Law*, 1: 289.

Muijen, M. (1996) 'Scare in the community: Britain in moral panic', in T. Heller, J. Reynolds, R. Gomm, R. Muston and S. Pattison (eds), *Mental Health Matters*, Milton Keynes: Open University Press, pp 143–55.

Murray, C.A. (1990) *The Emerging British Underclass* (Choice in Welfare), London: Institute of Economic Affairs.

Murray, R. (2017) 'Mistakes I have made in my research career', *Schizophrenia Bulletin*, 43: 253–6.

Nagel, T. (1970) *The Possibility of Altruism*, Princeton, NJ: Princeton University Press.

National Institute for Mental Health in England (2007) *Progress Report on the National Suicide Prevention Strategy*, Leeds: CSIP.

Nora, P. (1989) 'Between Memory and History: Les lieux de mémoire', *Representations*, 26 (Spring): 7–24.

Nye, R. (2003) 'The evolution of the concept of medicalisation in the twentieth century', *Journal of the History of Behavourial Sciences*, 39(2): 115–29.

O'Brien, A.J. (2014) 'Community treatment orders in New Zealand: regional variability and international comparisons', *Australasian Psychiatry*, 22(4): 352–6.

O'Brien, M. and Penna, S. (1998) *Theorising Welfare: Enlightenment and Modern Society*, London: Sage.

O'Farrell, M. (2006) *The Vanishing Act of Esme Lennox*, Dublin: Houghton Mifflin Harcourt.

Ornellas, A. (2014) 'Views of social workers on their role in mental health outpatient and community-based services', Doctoral dissertation, Stellenbosch University.

Ornellas, A. and Engelbrecht, L.K. (2018) 'The Life Esidimeni crisis: why a neoliberal agenda leaves no room for the mentally ill', *Social Work*, 54(3): 296–308.

Papeschi, R. (1985) 'The denial of the institution. A critical review of Franco Basaglia's writings', *The British Journal of Psychiatry*, 146(3): 247–54.

Park, R.E. (1967) 'The City: suggestions for the investigation of human behaviour in the urban environment' in R.E. Park and E.W. Burgess (eds), *The City*, Chicago: University of Chicago Press, pp 1–46.

Parr, H., Philo, C. and Burns, N. (2003) '"That awful place was home": Reflections on the Contested Meanings of Craig Dunain Asylum', *Scottish Geographical Journal*, 119(4): 341–60.

Parsons, A.E. (2018) *From Asylum to Prison: Deinstitutionalization and the Rise of Mass Incarceration After 1945*, Chapel Hill, NC: UNC Press.

Penrose, L.S. (1939) 'Mental disease and crime: outline of a comparative study of European statistics', *British Journal of Medical Psychology*, 18(1): 1–15.

Penrose, L.S. (1943) 'A note on the statistical relationship between mental deficiency and crime in the United States', *American Journal of Mental Deficiency*, 47: 462.

Philo, C. (1987) '"Fit localities for an asylum": the historical geography of the nineteenth-century "mad-business" in England as viewed through the pages of the Asylum Journal', *Journal of Historical Geography*, 13(4): 398–415.

Pilger, J. (1976) 'Dumped on the streets and in the slums: 5000 who need help', *Daily Mirror*, 12 January, studymore.org.uk/mhhtim. htm#1976

Platt, S., Stace, S. and Morrissey, J. (eds) (2017) *Dying From Inequality: Socioeconomic Disadvantage and Suicidal Behaviour*, London: Samaritans.

Pollitt, C. and Bouckaert, G. (2004) *Public Management Reform: A Comparative Analysis*, Oxford: Oxford University Press

Prins, H. (1993) *Big, Black and Dangerous. Report of the Committee of Inquiry into the Death in Broadmoor Hospital of Orville Blackwood and a Review of the Deaths of Two Other Afro-Caribbean Patients*, London: SHSA.

Prins, H. (1998) 'Inquiries after homicide in England and Wales', *Medicine, Science and the Law*, 38(3): 211–20.

Prins, H. (2004) 'Mental Health Inquiries – Views from the Chair', *Journal of Mental Health Law*, February: 7–15.

Prior, L. (2003) *Using Documents in Social Research*, London: Sage.

Rafferty, J.A., Abelson, J.M., Bryant, K. and Jackson, J.S. (2015) 'Discrimination', in M.T. Compton and R.S. Shim (eds), *The Social Determinants of Mental Health*, Washington DC: American Psychiatric Publishing.

Raphael, S. (2000) 'The deinstitutionalization of the mentally ill and growth in the US prison populations: 1971 to 1996', unpublished manuscript.

Raphael, S. and Stoll, M.A. (2013) *Why Are So Many Americans in Prison?*, Russell Sage Foundation.

Rawls, J. (1971) *A Theory of Justice*, Cambridge, MA: Harvard University Press.

Rehman, Z. (2016) 'How one indigenous reserve is coping with Canada's suicide crisis', *BuzzfeedNews*, 5 May, www.buzzfeednews.com/article/zrehman/why-are-indigenous-canadians-killing-themselves

Reiner, R. (2000) *The Politics of the Police* (3rd edn), Oxford: Oxford University Press.

Reith, M. (1998) 'Risk assessment and management: lessons from mental health inquiry reports', *Medicine, Science and the Law*, 38(3): 221–6.

Republic of South Africa (2004) *Mental Health Care Act* (17 of 2002), Pretoria: National Department of Health.

Republic of South Africa (2009) *National mental health policy framework and strategic plan 2013–2020*, Pretoria: National Department of Health.

Riley, G., Freeman, E., Laidlaw, J. and Pugh, D. (2011) '"A frightening experience": detainees' and carers' experiences of being detained under Section 136 of the Mental Health Act', *Medicine, Science and the Law*, 51(3): 164–9.

Ritchie, J., Dick, D. and Lingham, R. (1994) *Report of the Inquiry into the Care and Treatment of Christopher Clunis*, London: HMSO, North East Thames and South East Thames Regional Health Authorities.

Robb, B. (1967) *Sans Everything: A Case to Answer*, London: Thomas Nelson.

Rogers, A. and Faulkner, A. (1987) *A Place of Safety*, London: MIND Publications.

Rogers, A. and Pilgrim, D. (2014) *A Sociology of Mental Health and Illness*, Maidenhead: McGraw-Hill Education.

Rose, N. (1985) 'Unreasonable rights: Mental illness and the limits of the law', *Journal of Law and Society*, 12(2): 199–218.

Rose, N. (1994) 'Medicine, history and the present', in C. Jones and R. Porter (eds), *Reassessing Foucault: Power, Medicine and the Body*, London: Routledge, pp 48–72.

Rose, N. (1996) 'The death of the social? Re-figuring the territory of government', *International Journal of Human Resource Management*, 25(3): 327–56.

Rosenhan, D.L. (1975) 'On being sane in insane places', *Science*, 179(4070): 250–8.

Rothman, D. (2002) *The Discovery of the Asylum: Social Order and Disorder in the New Republic*, New York: Aldine de Gruyter.

Royal College of Nursing (2001) *Caring for Prisoners*, London: RCN.

Royal College of Psychiatrists (1996) *Report of the Confidential Inquiry into Homicides and Suicides by Mentally Disordered Offenders*, London: RCP.

Royal Commission (1926) *Report of Royal Commission on Lunacy and Mental Disorder*, London: HMSO.

Ryan, F. (2015) 'Death has become a part of Britain's benefits system', *The Guardian*, 17 August, www.theguardian.com/commentisfree/2015/aug/27/death-britains-benefits-system-fit-for-work-safety-net

Savage, M. (2015) *Social Class in the 21st Century*, London: Penguin.

Savage, M. (2017) 'Theresa May pledges mental health revolution will reduce detentions', *The Guardian*, 7 May, www.theguardian.com/politics/2017/may/07/theresa-may-pledges-mental-health-revolution-will-reduce-detentions

Sayce, L. (2000) *From Psychiatric Patient to Citizen: Overcoming Discrimination and Social Exclusion*, London: St Martin's Press.

Sayer, A. (2015) *Why We Can't Afford the Rich*, Bristol: Policy Press.

Schissel, B. (1997) *Blaming Children: Youth Crime, Moral Panics and the Politics of Hate*, Halifax, NS: Fernwood.

Scotland, Baroness, Kelly, H. and Devaux, M. (1998) *The Report of the Luke Warm Luke Mental Health Inquiry*, Volumes I and II, London: Lambeth, Lewisham and Southwark Health Authority

Scott, R.D. (1973) 'The treatment barrier part 1', *British Journal of Medical Psychology*, 46: 45–53.

Scull, A.T. (1977) 'Madness and segregative control: The rise of the insane asylum', *Social Problems*, 24(3): 337–51.

Scull, A. (1986) 'Mental patients and the community: A critical note', *International Journal of Law and Psychiatry*, 9(3): 383–92.

Scull, A. (1989) *Social Disorder*, Cambridge: Polity Press.

Scull, A. (1991) 'Psychiatry and its historians', *History of Psychiatry*, 2(7): 239–50.

Scull, A. (2014) *Madness in Civilization: A Cultural History of Insanity from the Bible to Freud, from the Madhouse to Modern Medicine*, Princeton: Princeton University Press.

Seddon, T. (2009) *Punishment and Madness: Governing Prisoners with Mental Health Problems*, London: Routledge-Cavendish.

Sedgwick, P. (1982) *Psychopolitics*, London: Pluto Press.

Sharpley, M., Hutchinson, G., Murray, R.M. and McKenzie, K. (2001) 'Understanding the excess of psychosis among the African-Caribbean population in England: review of current hypotheses', *The British Journal of Psychiatry*, 178(S40):s60–s68.

Shaw, J., Hunt, I.M., Flynn, S., Meehan, J., Robinson, J.O., Bickley, H., Parsons, R., McCann, K., Burns, J., Amos, T. and Kapur, N. (2006) 'Rates of mental disorder in people convicted of homicide: national clinical survey', *The British Journal of Psychiatry*, 188(2): 143–7.

Shen, G.C. and Snowden, L.R. (2014) 'Institutionalization of deinstitutionalization: A cross-national analysis of mental health system reform', *International Journal of Mental Health Systems*, 8(47): 1–23.

Sheppard, D. (1995) *Learning the Lesson: Mental Health Enquiry Reports Published in England and Wales Between 1969–1994 and Their Recommendations for Improving Practice*, London: Zito Trust

Sheppard, D. (1998) *Learning the Lessons*, London: Zito Trust.

Shim, R., Koplan, C., Langheim, F.J.P., Manseau, M.W., Powers, R.A. and Compton, M.T. (2014) 'The social determinants of mental health: An overview and call to action', *Psychiatric Annals*, 44: 22–6.

Sibley, D. (1995) *Geographies of Exclusion: Society and Difference in the West*, London: Routledge.

Silva, M., Loureiro, A. and Cardoso, G. (2016) 'Social determinants of mental health: A review of the evidence', *European Journal of Psychiatry*, 30: 259–92.

Simmel, G. (2004) 'The Stranger', in C. Jenlis (ed), *Urban Culture and Critical Concepts in Literary and Cultural Studies*, Volume III, London: Routledge, pp 73–7.

Simon, J. (2007) *Governing Through Crime: How the War on Crime Transformed American Democracy and Created a Culture of Fear*, Oxford: Oxford University Press.

Simon, J. (2014) 'Law's violence, the strong state, and the crisis of mass imprisonment (for Stuart Hall)', *Wake Forest Law Review*, 49: 649.

Simon, J. and Rosenbaum, S. (2015) 'Dignifying madness: rethinking commitment law in an age of mass incarceration', *University of Miami Law Review*, 70(1): 1–52.

Singleton, N., Meltzer, H. and Gatward, R. (1998) *Psychiatric Morbidity Among Prisoners in England and Wales*, London: Office for National Statistics.

Skelcher, C. (2000) 'Changing images of the state: overloaded, hollowed-out, congested', *Public Policy and Administration*, 15(3): 3–19.

Slater, T. (2009) 'Ghettos' and 'Anti-urbanism', in R. Kitchin and N. Thrift (eds), *The International Encyclopaedia of Human Geography*, London: Elsevier.

Slater, T. (2018) 'The invention of the "sink estate": Consequential categorisation and the UK housing crisis', *The Sociological Review*, 66(4): 877–97.

Soja, E.W. (1996) *Thirdspace: Journeys to Los Angeles and other Real-Imagined Places*, Cambridge, MA: Blackwell.

Somers, M. (2008) *Genealogies of Citizenship. Markets, Statelessness and the Right to Have Rights*, Cambridge: Cambridge University Press.

Standing, G. (2011) *The Precariat: The New Dangerous Class*, London: Bloomsbury.

Stanley, N. and Manthorpe, J. (2001) 'Reading mental health inquiries: Messages for social work', *Journal of Social Work*, 1(1): 77–99.

Steel, J., Thornicroft, G., Birmingham, L., Brooker, C., Mills, A., Harty, M. and Shaw, J. (2007) 'Prison mental health inreach services', *The British Journal of Psychiatry*, 190(5): 373–4.

Stone, L. (1982) 'An exchange with Michel Foucault', *New York Review of Books*, 31 March.

Stuckler, D. and Basu, S. (2013) *The Body Economic: Why Austerity Kills*, New York: Basic Books.

Subramanian, R. and Shames, A. (2013) *Sentencing and Prison Practices in Germany and the Netherlands: Implications for the United States*, New York: Vera Institute of Justice.

Swinson, N., Flynn, S.M., While, D., Roscoe, A., Kapur, N., Appleby, L. and Shaw, J. (2011) 'Trends in rates of mental illness in homicide perpetrators', *The British Journal of Psychiatry*, 198(6): 485–9.

Szasz, T. (1963) *Law, Liberty and Psychiatry*, New York: Macmillan.

Szasz, T. (1971) *The Manufacture of Madness*, London: Routledge and Kegan Paul.

Szasz, T. (1992) 'The myth of mental illness', in R. Miller (ed), *The Restoration of Dialogue: Readings in the Philosophy of Clinical Psychology*, Washington: American Psychological Association.

Szasz, T. (1995) 'Idleness and lawlessness in the therapeutic state', *Society*, 32(4): 31–35.

Szmukler, G. (2000) 'Homicide inquiries: what sense do they make?' *Psychiatric Bulletin*, 24(1): 6–10.

Szmukler, G. (2018) *Men in White Coats: Treatment under Coercion*, Oxford: Oxford University Press.

Talbot, J.A. (2004) 'Deinstitutionalization: Avoiding the disasters of the past', *Psychiatric Services*, 55(10): 1112–15.

Taylor, C. (2003) *Modern Social Imaginaries*, Durham, NC: Duke University Press.

Taylor, P.J. and Gunn, J. (1999) 'Homicides by people with mental illness: myth and reality', *British Journal of Psychiatry*, 174: 9–14.

Taylor-Gooby, P. (2012) 'Root and branch restructuring to achieve major cuts: The social policy programme of the 2010 UK coalition government', *Social Policy & Administration*, 46(1): 61–82.

Teplin, L.A. (1984) 'Criminalizing mental disorder: the comparative arrest rate of the mentally ill', *American Psychologist*, 39(7): 794.

Todd, S. (2015) *The People: The Rise and Fall of the Working Class, 1910–2010*, London: John Murray.

Tonnies, E. (1955) *Community and Society*, London: Routledge and Kegan Paul.

Topor, A. and Ljungqvist, I. (2017) 'Money, social relationships and the sense of self: The consequences of an improved financial situation for persons suffering from serious mental illness', *Community Mental Health Journal*, 53: 823–31.

Torrey, E.F. (1988) *Nowhere to go: The tragic odyssey of the homeless mentally ill*, New York: Harper & Row.

Torrey, E.F. (1997) *Out of the Shadows: Confronting America's Mental Illness Crisis*, New York: John Wiley.

Torrey, E.F (1998) *Nowhere to Go: The Tragic Odyssey of the Homeless Mentally Ill*, New York: Harper & Row.

Torrey, E.F. (2010) 'Documenting the failure of deinstitutionalization', *Psychiatry*, 73(2): 122–4.

Torrey, E.F., Kennard, A.D., Eslinger, D., Lamb, R. and Pavle, J. (2010) *More Mentally Ill Persons are in Jails and Prisons than Hospitals: A Survey of the States*, Arlington, VA: Treatment Advocacy Center.

Tuan, Y.F. (1979) 'Space and place: humanistic perspective', in S. Gale and G. Olsson (eds), *Philosophy in Geography*, Dordrecht: Springer, pp 387–427.

Turner. T and Colombo A. (2008) 'Risk', in R. Tummey and T. Turner (eds), *Critical Issues in Mental Health*, Basingstoke: Palgrave Macmillan.

Tyler, I. (2013) *Revolting Subjects: Social Abjection and Resistance in Neoliberal Britain*, London: Zed Books.

United Nations General Assembly (1948) *Universal Declaration of Human Rights*, UN General Assembly.

Van der Velde, M. (2016) *Abandoned Asylums*, Paris: Jonglez Publishing.

Vergunst, F., Rugkåsa, J., Koshiaris, C., Simon, J. and Burns, T. (2017) 'Community treatment orders and social outcomes for patients with psychosis: a 48-month follow-up study', *Social Psychiatry and Psychiatric Epidemiology*, 52(11): 1375–84.

Wacquant, L. (2005) 'Race as civic felony', *International Social Science Journal*, 57(183): 127–142.

Wacquant, L. (2007) 'Territorial stigmatization in the age of advanced marginality', *Thesis Eleven*, 91: 66–77.

Wacquant, L. (2008a) 'Ghettos and anti-ghettos: An anatomy of the new urban poverty', *Thesis Eleven,* 94: 113–18.

Wacquant, L. (2008b) *Urban Outcasts: A Comparative Sociology of Advanced Marginality*, Cambridge: Polity Press.

Wacquant, L. (2009a) *Prisons of Poverty*, Minneapolis, MN: University of Minnesota Press.

Wacquant, L. (2009b) *Punishing the Poor: The Neoliberal Government of Social Insecurity*, Durham, NC: Duke University Press.

Wacquant, L. (2010) 'Urban desolation and symbolic denigration in the hyperghetto', *Social Psychology Quarterly*, 73(3): 215–219.

Wacquant, L. (2013) 'The wedding of workfare and prisonfare in the 21st century: responses to critics and commentators', in P. Squires and J. Lea (eds), *Criminalisation and Advanced Marginality: Critically Exploring the Work of Loïc Wacquant*, Bristol: Policy Press, pp 243–58.

Wacquant, L. (2016) 'Revisiting territories of relegation: Class, ethnicity and state in the making of advanced marginality', *Urban Studies*, 53(6): 1077–88.

Walmsley, R. (2015) *World Female Imprisonment List* (3rd edn), https://www.prisonstudies.org/search/node/world%20female%20 imprisonment https://www.prisonstudies.org/

Warden, J. (1998) 'England abandons care in the community for the mentally ill', *BMJ*, 317(1611).

Warner, J. (2006) 'Inquiry reports as active texts and their function in relation to professional practice in mental health', *Health, Risk & Society*, 8(3): 223–37.

Warner, J. (2015) *The Emotional Politics of Social Work and Child Protection*, Bristol: Policy Press.

Weissmann, G. (1982) 'Foucault and the bag lady', *Hospital Practice*, 17(8): 28–39.

Welshman, J. (2013) *Underclass: A History of the Excluded Since 1880*, London: Bloomsbury.

Wheen, F. (2009) *Strange Days Indeed: The Golden Age of Paranoia*, London: Fourth Estate.

World Health Organization (WHO) (2005) *WHO Resource Book on Mental Health, Human Rights and Legislation*, Geneva: World Health Organisation.

WHO (2008) *Trencin statement on prisons and mental health*, Copenhagen: World Health Organization, Regional Office for Europe, www.euro.who.int/en/health-topics/health-determinants/prisons-and-health/publications/2007/trencin-statement-on-prisons-and-mental-health

WHO (2014) *Social determinants of mental health*, Geneva: World Health Organisation, https://www.who.int/mental_health/publications/gulbenkian_paper_social_determinants_of_mental_health/en/

Wilkinson, R. and Pickett, K. (2010) *The Spirit Level: Why Equality is Better for Everyone*, London: Penguin.

Wilkinson, R. and Pickett, K. (2017) 'The enemy between us: The psychological and social costs of inequality', *European Journal of Social Psychology*, 47(1): 11–24.

Wilkinson, R. and Pickett, K. (2018) *The Inner Level: How More Equal Societies Reduce Stress, Restore Sanity and Improve Everyone's Well-being*, London: Penguin.

Williams, R. (2014) *Keywords: A Vocabulary of Culture and Society*, Oxford: Oxford University Press.

Winerup, M. (1999) 'Bedlam on the streets', *New York Times*, 23 May, www.nytimes.com/1999/05/23/magazine/bedlam-on-the-streets.html

Wing, J. (1962) 'Institutionalism in mental hospitals', *British Journal of Social and Clinical Psychology*, 1: 38–51

Wing, J. (1978) *Reasoning about Madness*, Oxford: Oxford University Press.

Wolff, N. (2005) 'Community reintegration of prisoners with mental illness: a social investment perspective', *International Journal of Law and Psychiatry*, 28: 43–58.

Wood, J., Swanson, J., Burris, S. and Gilbert, A. (2011) *Police Interventions with Persons Affected by Mental Illnesses: A Critical Review of Global Thinking and Practice*, New Brunswick, NJ: Center for Behavioral Health Services & Criminal Justice Research, Rutgers University.

Woolf, Lord Chief Justice (1991) *Prison Disturbances: April 1990*, Cm. 1456, London: HMSO.

Yar, M. and Penna, S. (2004) 'Between positivism and post-modernity? Critical reflections on Jock Young's *The Exclusive Society*', *British Journal of Criminology*, 44: 533–49.

Young, H. (2013) *One of Us* (final edn), London: Pan Books.

Young, J. (1999) *The Exclusive Society: Social Exclusion, Crime and Difference in Late Modernity*, London: Sage.

1990 Trust (2010) *The Price of Race Inequality: The Black Manifesto*, London: 1990 Trust.

Index